SERIES 2
PROVISION

Preferred Responses in Ophthalmology

A Self-Assessment Program

Volume I: Questions

Gregory L. Skuta, MD
Executive Editor

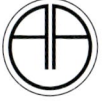
American Academy of Ophthalmology

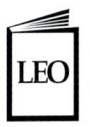
Lifelong Education for the Ophthalmologist

American Academy of Ophthalmology
655 Beach Street, P.O. Box 7424
San Francisco, CA 94120-7424

Academy Staff

Kathryn A. Hecht, EdD, Vice President, Clinical Education

Programs Department
William M. Hering, PhD, Director, Programs Department
Stephen Moore, PhD, Self-Assessment Program Manager

Publications Department
Hal Straus, Director, Publications Department
Margaret Petela, Managing Editor, Special Projects
Lisa Bogle, Production Manager
Beth T. Berkelhammer, Production Assistant
Rachel Griener, Administrative Assistant

Designed by Mark Ong, Side by Side Studios

This program is supported in part by a grant from Otsuka America Pharmaceutical, Inc.

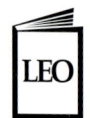

ProVision: Preferred Responses in Ophthalmology, Series 2, is one component in the Lifelong Education for the Ophthalmologist (LEO) framework, which assists members in planning their continuing medical education. LEO includes an array of clinical education products and programs that members may select to form individualized, self-directed learning plans for updating their clinical knowledge. Active members and fellows who use LEO components may accumulate sufficient CME credits to earn the LEO Award. Contact the Academy's Clinical Education Division for further information on LEO.

This CME activity was planned and produced in accordance with the ACCME Essentials.

Because diagnostic, therapeutic, and practice recommendations (hereinafter "recommendations") may have changed since the publication of this book, because such recommendations cannot be considered absolute or universal in their application, and because the publication process contains the potential for error, the American Academy of Ophthalmology strongly advises that the recommendations in this book be verified, prior to use, with information included in the manufacturers' package inserts or provided by an independent source and be considered in light of a particular patient's clinical condition and history. Caution is especially urged when using new or infrequently used drugs. Including all indications, contraindications, side effects, and alternative agents for each drug or treatment is beyond the scope of this book.

The Academy disclaims responsibility and liability for any and all adverse medical or legal effects, including personal, bodily, property, or business injury, and for damages or loss of any kind whatsoever, resulting directly or indirectly, whether from negligence or otherwise, from the use of the recommendations or other information in this book, from any undetected printing errors or recommendation errors, or from textual misunderstandings by the reader. The ultimate arbiter of any diagnostic or therapeutic decision remains the individual physician's judgment.

Reference to certain drugs, instruments, and other products in this publication is made for illustrative purposes only and is not intended to constitute an endorsement of such drugs, instruments, and other products.

ISBN 1-56055-031-7

Copyright © 1996 American Academy of Ophthalmology®
All rights reserved.

97 98 99 00   4 3 2 1

Contents

Acknowledgments	v
Preface	vii
Introduction: *ProVision* and Lifelong Education for the Ophthalmologist (LEO)	ix
How to Use *ProVision* Series 2	xi

SECTION ONE
Glaucoma   1

SECTION TWO
External Disease and Cornea   19

SECTION THREE
Cataract and Anterior Segment Surgery   39

SECTION FOUR
Neuro-Ophthalmology   59

SECTION FIVE
Orbit and Ophthalmic Plastic Surgery   81

SECTION SIX
Pediatric Ophthalmology and Strabismus   101

SECTION SEVEN
Retina and Vitreous   123

SECTION EIGHT
Optics, Refraction, Contact Lens, and Visual Rehabilitation   149

Acknowledgments

The American Academy of Ophthalmology gratefully acknowledges the contributions of numerous individuals in the development of this program, especially the members of the Self-Assessment Committee.

Self-Assessment Committee

Gregory L. Skuta, MD, *Chair*
Oklahoma City, Oklahoma

Keith D. Carter, MD
Iowa City, Iowa

Susan G. Elner, MD
Ann Arbor, Michigan

Larry P. Frohman, MD
Newark, New Jersey

Edward K. Isbey, Jr, MD
Asheville, North Carolina

Ronald V. Keech, MD
Iowa City, Iowa

Stephen S. Lane, MD
St. Paul, Minnesota

Mark J. Mannis, MD
Sacramento, California

Edward J. Rockwood, MD
Cleveland, Ohio

Contributors

Section 1
Edward J. Rockwood, MD; Beverly C. Forcier, MD; Kathleen A. Lamping, MD
Reviewers: L. Jay Katz, MD; Rebecca K. Morgan, MD

Section 2
Mark J. Mannis, MD
Reviewers: Mark L. McDermott, MD; Michael P. Vrabec, MD

Section 3
Stephen S. Lane, MD; James A. Davison, MD; Harry B. Grabow, MD; Thomas D. Lindquist, MD, PhD; Scott M. MacRae, MD; Samuel Masket, MD; James J. Salz, MD; Theodore P. Werblin, MD, PhD
Reviewers: Douglas D. Koch, MD; Alan Sugar, MD

Section 4
Larry P. Frohman, MD; Anthony C. Arnold, MD; Mark J. Kupersmith, MD; Jonathan D. Trobe, MD
Reviewers: Roy W. Beck, MD; Nancy J. Newman, MD; Jonathan D. Trobe, MD; Floyd A. Warren, MD

Section 5
Keith D. Carter, MD; Ronan M. Conlon, MD, FRCSC; Gene R. Howard, MD; Jeffrey A. Nerad, MD; John J. Woog, MD
Reviewers: George B. Bartley, MD; Robert G. Small, MD

Section 6
Ronald V. Keech, MD; Laurie E. Christiansen, MD; Arlene V. Drack, MD; Christina P. Johnson, MD; David A. Johnson, MD, PhD; G. Frank Judisch, MD; Scott R. Lambert, MD; P. David Reese, MD; Terry L. Schwartz, MD; Sarah J. Stair, MD; Edwin M. Stone, MD, PhD
Reviewers: Steven M. Archer, MD; Mark H. Scott, MD

Section 7
Susan G. Elner, MD; Barbara A. Blodi, MD; Mark W. Johnson, MD; Michael J. Shapiro, MD; Paul A. Sieving, MD, PhD; Andrew K. Vine, MD
Reviewers: Maryanna Destro, MD; Dennis P. Han, MD

Section 8
J. Wayne Beaton, MD; Robert M. Christiansen, MD; Donald C. Fletcher, MD; David L. Guyton, MD; Jack T. Holladay, MD; Jeffrey T. Liegner, MD; Jean Ann Vickery, FCLSA
Reviewers: Cynthia A. Bradford, MD; Stephen R. Russell, MD

PREFACE

The American Academy of Ophthalmology is pleased to offer Series 2 of *ProVision: Preferred Responses in Ophthalmology*. Participation in *ProVision* Series 1, which was released late in 1992, has greatly exceeded original projections, requiring a second printing after the program's second year. In a 1993 survey of *ProVision* Series 1 users, more than 95 percent of respondents either agreed or strongly agreed that *ProVision* had effectively challenged, assessed, and instructed them, and 98 percent indicated that they would recommend *ProVision* to a colleague.

Given the success of *ProVision* Series 1, we are particularly indebted to Dr Thomas A. Weingeist, who, as the first chair of the Self-Assessment Committee and executive editor of *ProVision* Series 1, developed the objectives and organization of this program. Members of the Self-Assessment Committee and the numerous other contributors and formal reviewers for *ProVision* Series 2 listed in the Acknowledgments have volunteered an enormous amount of time and meticulous effort to ensure the quality of this educational product. In addition, the Academy's Practicing Ophthalmologists Advisory Committee on Education and its chair, Dr Hal D. Balyeat, have provided valuable feedback during the preparation of *ProVision* Series 2. As always, the dedication of the Academy staff to successful completion of this project has been critical. Special thanks are due to Stephen Moore, Self-Assessment Program Manager; Margaret Petela, Managing Editor; and Lisa Bogle, Production Manager.

In preparing *ProVision: Preferred Responses in Ophthalmology* Series 2, the committee carefully considered suggestions for improvements that came from users of Series 1, leading clinicians, and professional educators. In keeping with these suggestions, the committee increased the number of sections from seven to eight, each with 50 questions, and included many more color photographs and clinical images. In developing questions and discussions, the committee emphasized areas likely to be encountered by a contemporary comprehensive ophthalmologist, such as phacoemulsification, refractive surgery, infectious disease, ocular oncology, uveitis, and systemic disease.

Although Series 2 offers significant improvements, Series 1 is in no way outdated or superseded; it continues to be the excellent assessment instrument that it always has been. The two products comprise different questions and emphasize different clinical topics. Therefore, practitioners who have not already done so are encouraged to broaden the scope of their self-assessment by also completing *ProVision* Series 1.

All ophthalmologists certified by the American Board of Ophthalmology in 1992 and thereafter will require renewal of their certification every ten years. Time-limited certification, together with other challenges in our profession, makes developing a self-directed lifelong learning program a logical and vital step for all ophthalmologists. We hope that you will find participation in *ProVision* Series 2 a meaningful experience that, together with other elements of the LEO framework, will satisfy your needs for personal assessment and learning and, most importantly, result in the highest possible quality of care for your patients.

Gregory L. Skuta, MD
Oklahoma City, Oklahoma

INTRODUCTION

ProVision and Lifelong Education for the Ophthalmologist (LEO)

In this era of tremendous change in the field of medicine, it is essential for every ophthalmologist to develop a self-directed lifelong learning program. With this in mind, Academy President Dr Ronald Smith officially launched "Lifelong Education for the Ophthalmologist" (LEO) at the 1994 Annual Meeting. The LEO framework encompasses an array of continuing medical education products and programs organized to help ophthalmologists formulate and implement individualized learning plans that address their personal educational goals:

- All ophthalmologists may develop LEO plans to help them become more comprehensive in their practices.
- Subspecialists may develop LEO plans to update their knowledge outside their own subspecialties.
- Members preparing to meet the requirements of certification renewal or managed care groups may develop LEO plans to organize and focus their educational efforts.

Within the LEO framework, the field of ophthalmology is divided into ten areas:

1. Glaucoma
2. Cataract and Anterior Segment Surgery
3. Cornea, External Disease, and Anterior Segment Trauma
4. Ocular Oncology
5. Neuro-Ophthalmology
6. Orbit and Ophthalmic Plastic Surgery
7. Pediatric Ophthalmology and Strabismus
8. Retina, Vitreous, and Posterior Segment Trauma
9. Uveitis and General Medicine
10. Refraction, Contact Lens, and Visual Rehabilitation

Ten Clinical Topic Updates, one for each of these areas, are the latest offerings from LEO. Each is designed to give an overview of its topic, focusing on advances made in the last 5 to 10 years. The Clinical Topic Updates serve as entry points into the LEO framework by assisting ophthalmologists in determining the topics and resources to incorporate in their LEO plans. Call or write the Academy or consult the Academy catalog for availability of the Clinical Topic Updates.

As a tool for assessing ophthalmic knowledge and identifying learning needs, *ProVision* complements the Clinical Topic Updates and serves as another entry point into the LEO framework. Although *ProVision* cannot offer a complete assessment of a practitioner's knowledge and skill, it can indicate areas in which additional study may be warranted. The subspecialty sections in *ProVision* differ somewhat from the ten LEO topics. The developers of Series 2 retained the seven sections from Series 1 and added an eighth, "Optics, Refraction, Contact Lens, and Visual Rehabilitation." Although two of the LEO topics, "Ocular Oncology" and "Uveitis and General Medicine," do not appear as separate sections in Series 2, questions on these topics are included, where appropriate, throughout.

The Academy will continue to develop new LEO products and programs to keep pace with the changing needs of Academy members. LEO Update Courses will be offered during the Annual Meeting and at other times. A LEO project under development is *ProVision Interactive,* a multimedia self-assessment program on CD-ROM. Motion video, audio, computer graphics, and enhanced still photographs will combine to create an interactive environment that realistically simulates patient–physician encounters. Please contact the Academy for information about the availability of these programs.

HOW TO USE
PROVISION SERIES 2

Components and Contents

ProVision consists of two text volumes and one workbook. Volume I, "Questions," provides 50 multiple-choice test items in each of eight sections. The questions in *ProVision* require recall and application of medical knowledge, as well as clinical decision making and judgment. Many of the questions are presented as case studies, providing patient history, symptoms and signs, and test results, including relevant photographs and illustrations. Strong emphasis is placed on awareness of new clinical approaches to the diagnosis and treatment of eye diseases and disorders.

Volume II, "Discussions," duplicates every question and clinical image from Volume I, provides a discussion of each question, and indicates the preferred response. In the discussions, recognized experts in the field explain the clinical and scientific reasons for choosing the preferred response, and give numerous citations to the literature. Lists of all references and pertinent Academy resources are provided at the end of each section in Volume II.

Going beyond standard assessment, *ProVision* emphasizes learning by providing instructional feedback. The term "preferred response" is used instead of "correct answer" to acknowledge the ongoing debate on some clinical points. Because we have included controversial topics, you may not always agree with the preferred response or discussion. The discussions and the preferred responses are based on the information presented in the questions and should not be construed as excluding other acceptable practices.

The Workbook contains

- A Worksheet for recording your responses
- The Program Evaluation and CME Credit Report
- The Self-Evaluation Learning Plan
- A Machine-Scorable Answer Sheet
- The Worksheet Answer Key for self-scoring

The Self-Evaluation Learning Plan and the Machine-Scorable Answer Sheet are provided as alternative ways to obtain Continuing Medical Education credit for *ProVision* and are explained below.

Recommended Approach

The Academy recommends that you work through *ProVision* one section at a time. You need not complete the sections in the order presented, but you should answer all questions for one section in Volume I before reviewing the discussions and preferred responses for that section in Volume II. For maximum benefit, you should read the discussion for every question—whether you chose the preferred response or not—because any discussion may contain some information that is new to you or that relates to another question or discussion. You should record and tally your responses, using the Worksheet and Worksheet Answer Key in the Workbook, and note the specific clinical points made in the discussions that you did not know or with which you disagree. This is the best way for you to identify strengths as well as areas needing further study. (Also please see the section below entitled "Establishing Your Educational Needs.") The Academy recommends that you complete all eight sections, giving special attention to those areas that are *not* a part of your everyday practice. Allow between 3 and 4 hours to complete an entire section (both volumes) in one sitting.

It is also possible to complete all the questions in Volume I before going on to Volume II. If you choose this approach, you may need to set aside approximately 12 hours for Volume I and 16 hours to review the discussions and preferred responses in Volume II. You may instead choose to work through Volume II alone, responding to a question, reading the corresponding discussion, and checking the preferred response before moving to the next question. With this approach, however, you are likely to overestimate your proficiency. Therefore, you should choose this alternative only if you are interested in *ProVision* solely as an educational program. To conduct the most effective self-assessment and to learn the most from the discussions, the Academy encourages you to complete the program as recommended.

Establishing Your Educational Needs

- The questions and discussions in *ProVision* represent only a sample from a larger field of knowledge. Take this into consideration when using *ProVision* to identify areas for further study.
- Do not limit your study solely to those clinical points made in the discussions. Rather, focus on the broader clinical areas of which those points are a part.
- Exercise caution in gauging your knowledge even on questions for which your answer did agree with the preferred response. Verify that your reasoning was clinically valid by studying the discussions for those questions too, not just for the ones you missed.
- The sections are not all equal in difficulty. For this reason, it is not possible to provide an objective performance standard or "passing grade" for any of the sections. Begin establishing your educational needs with any section or sections on which you scored substantially lower than on the other sections—say 25 percent lower.
- Make use of the two lists provided at the end of each section in Volume II. The first is a list of the references cited in support of the specific clinical points made in the discussions themselves. The second is a list of Academy educational resources.
- One self-assessment program cannot identify all areas in which you need more study. *ProVision* Series 1 and the Clinical Topic Updates are useful in identifying other areas needing further study.

Obtaining CME Credit

The American Academy of Ophthalmology is accredited to sponsor Continuing Medical Education (CME) for physicians by the Accreditation Council for Continuing Medical Education. The Academy designates up to 28 Category 1 CME credit hours for participation in *ProVision* Series 2, allowing one credit hour for every hour you spend.

Active members or fellows who participate in LEO may earn the LEO Continuing Education Recognition Award. To qualify, participants must complete 150 hours of Academy-sponsored Category 1 CME credits within a 3-year period, including participation in at least one Academy Annual Meeting or completion of a *ProVision* program. Through an agreement of reciprocity, all LEO Award recipients will be eligible for the American Medical Association's Standard Physician Recognition Award (PRA) certificate.

To apply for your *ProVision* CME credit, you must complete and send to the Academy two forms found in the *ProVision* Workbook:

- The Program Evaluation and CME Credit Report *(both sides)*

Plus one of the following two forms:

- OPTION 1: The Machine-Scorable Answer Sheet *(not the self-scoring Worksheet)*
- OPTION 2: The Self-Evaluation Learning Plan

If you choose to complete the Machine-Scorable Answer Sheet, you will receive a letter from the Academy that gives your scores, the average scores of your peers who also chose Option 1, and some general information about how to interpret your scores. These letters are sent out quarterly. Strict procedures are maintained to ensure the absolute confidentiality of the letters themselves and all information used to generate them. Because the answer sheet is scored by machine, *you must send in the original; photocopies cannot be processed.* Also, please fill in the bubbles completely with blue ink, black ink, or a No. 2 pencil. *Do not send the self-scoring Worksheet for machine scoring.*

If you choose to complete the Self-Evaluation Learning Plan (Option 2), you will formulate specific learning objectives and identify resources and activities that will allow you to accomplish those objectives. There will be no further followup from the Academy.

Although you would receive no additional CME credit for doing so, you may wish to complete both Option 1 and Option 2. You are encouraged also to consider earning additional CME through other Academy publications, programs, and courses, including the courses and seminars available at the Academy's Annual Meeting.

Regardless of the CME credit option you choose, the Academy requires that you also complete the Program Evaluation and CME Credit Report. The Program Evaluation is part of the CME requirement because it is vitally important for the Academy to know your level of satisfaction with *ProVision. Even if you are not applying for CME credit, please fill out the Program Evaluation portion of the form and return it to the Academy.* All evaluation information is processed anonymously. Your candid opinions and comments will help the Academy improve future *ProVision* programs.

SECTION ONE
GLAUCOMA

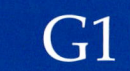 Five weeks after a trabeculectomy, a patient presents with a low, scarred bleb and intraocular pressure of 44 mm Hg (see the figure). After instituting therapy with a topical beta blocker, oral carbonic anhydrase inhibitor, and ocular digital massage, the intraocular pressure is 34 mm Hg.

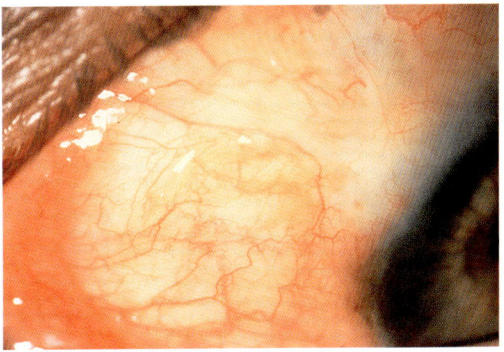

The *most* appropriate next step would be to

a. give subconjunctival 5-fluorouracil injections
b. perform Nd:YAG laser surgery to the internal aspect of the sclerostomy
c. needle the bleb
d. repeat trabeculectomy at a new operative site, using antifibrotic therapy

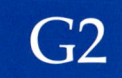 A patient complains of itching, redness, and scaling of the eyelids and periorbital skin (see the figure, part A). Conjunctival findings are shown in part B of the figure. He is on topical timolol, dipivefrin, and pilocarpine as well as oral acetazolamide for glaucoma.

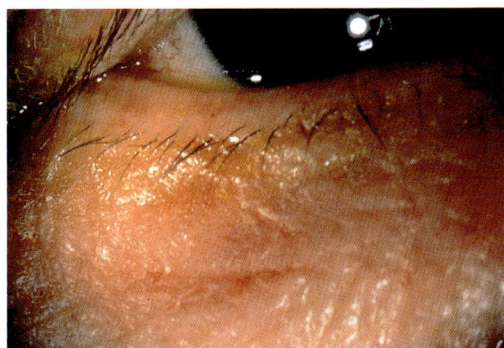
A

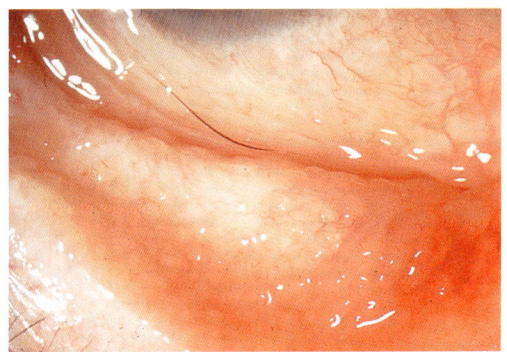
B

Which of the following actions will *most* likely resolve this problem?

a. discontinue timolol
b. discontinue dipivefrin
c. discontinue pilocarpine
d. prescribe topical dexamethasone ointment

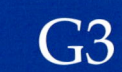

All of the following can cause a superior visual field defect in automated threshold perimetry *except*

a. glaucoma
b. ptosis
c. lens rim artifact
d. high false-positive rate

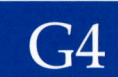

Assuming equal transmission and absorption of laser energy, which time and power setting below would provide energy equal to that delivered by an argon laser with settings of 0.1 sec duration and 500 mW power?

a. 0.05 sec; 2 W
b. 0.02 sec; 1 W
c. 0.02 sec; 2.5 W
d. 1 sec; 5 W

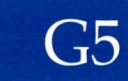

A 55-year-old man with no previous ocular laser or surgical therapy has advanced glaucomatous visual field loss (see the figure) and cupping. His current intraocular pressure is 37 mm Hg on a beta blocker and pilocarpine. An oral carbonic anhydrase inhibitor was previously tried but was discontinued because the patient complained of malaise and fatigue.

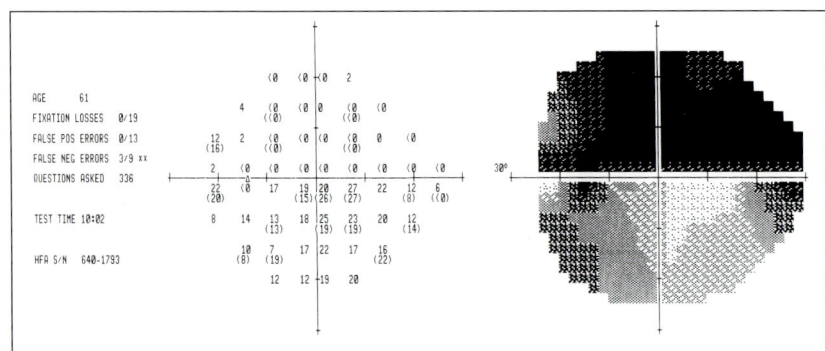

The next therapeutic step would be to

a. begin a second trial of oral carbonic anhydrase inhibitor and reinforce the need for compliance to prevent visual loss
b. switch from pilocarpine to carbachol to see if intraocular pressure control improved
c. perform laser trabeculoplasty
d. perform trabeculectomy

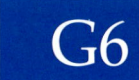 A patient with primary open-angle glaucoma underwent trabeculectomy. On the first postoperative day, the visual acuity corrects to 20/80, the bleb is almost flat, the anterior chamber is shallow (see the figure), and the intraocular pressure is 1 mm Hg.

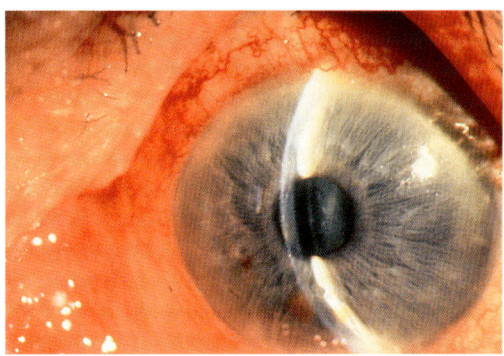

The *most* likely problem is

a. early failure of bleb with scarring at episcleral surface
b. ciliary body shutdown
c. bleb leak
d. aqueous misdirection (malignant or ciliary-block glaucoma)

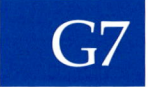 Medical management of glaucoma associated with inflammatory ocular disease (uveitis) and active intraocular inflammation could include all of the following *except*

a. pilocarpine
b. beta blocker
c. topical corticosteroid
d. cholinergic antagonist (cycloplegic agent)

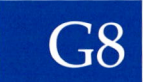 Which of the following would be the weakest indication for a combined cataract extraction and trabeculectomy in a patient with glaucoma and a visually significant cataract?

a. well-controlled glaucoma (intraocular pressure 13 mm Hg) on a topical beta blocker, miotic agent, and oral carbonic anhydrase inhibitor
b. glaucoma controlled with one medication in an eye with advanced glaucomatous visual field loss
c. an eye with previous trabeculectomy and with intraocular pressure of 18 mm Hg on a beta blocker and miotic agent
d. an eye with a previous history of acute angle-closure glaucoma, treated with laser iridotomy, and now with an intraocular pressure of 17 mm Hg on no medication and with no peripheral anterior synechiae

G9 The weakest indication for antifibrotic therapy in conjunction with glaucoma filtering surgery would be

a. primary trabeculectomy and exfoliation syndrome (pseudoexfoliation) glaucoma
b. neovascular glaucoma
c. glaucoma in pseudophakia
d. previously failed glaucoma filtering surgery

G10 All of the following are commonly seen in primary infantile glaucoma *except*

a. increased corneal diameter
b. myopia
c. prominent, anteriorly displaced Schwalbe's line
d. breaks in Descemet's membrane

G11 The *most* common reason for long-term visual loss in primary infantile glaucoma is

a. amblyopia
b. corneal edema
c. corneal scarring
d. glaucomatous optic nerve damage

G12 All of the following are risk factors for failure after glaucoma filtering surgery *except*

a. pigmentary dispersion
b. iris neovascularization
c. aphakia
d. uveitis

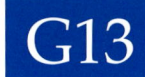

A patient presents 2 years after glaucoma filtering surgery with purulent discharge and endophthalmitis. Which of the following is the *most* likely causative organism?

a. *Staphylococcus epidermidis*
b. *Streptococcus pneumoniae*
c. *Pseudomonas aeruginosa*
d. *Propionibacterium acnes*

A generalized depression of all thresholds is shown on the central field automated perimetric test below.

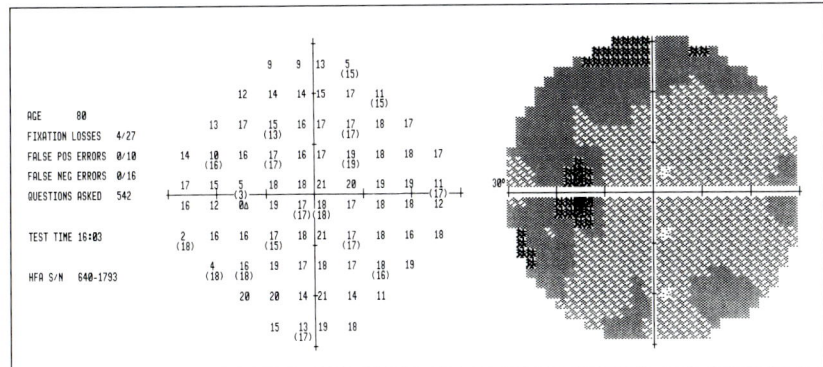

This finding could be a result of any of the following *except*

a. cataract
b. lens rim artifact
c. miotic agent
d. inaccurate optical correction for near

G15 Of the visual field defects shown, which would be *least* suggestive of glaucoma?

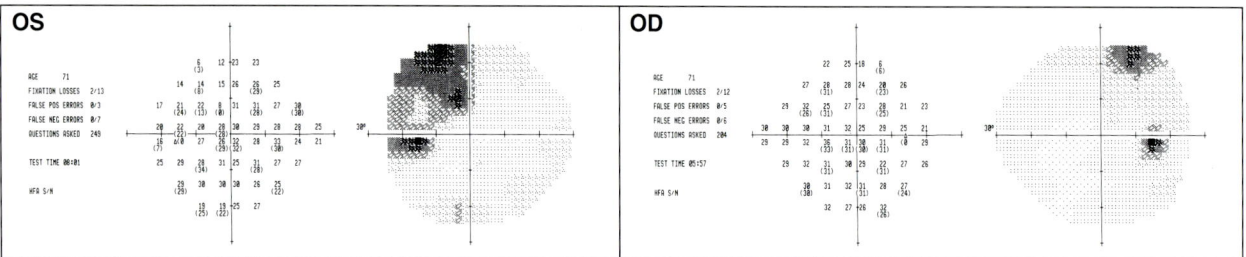

Figure A

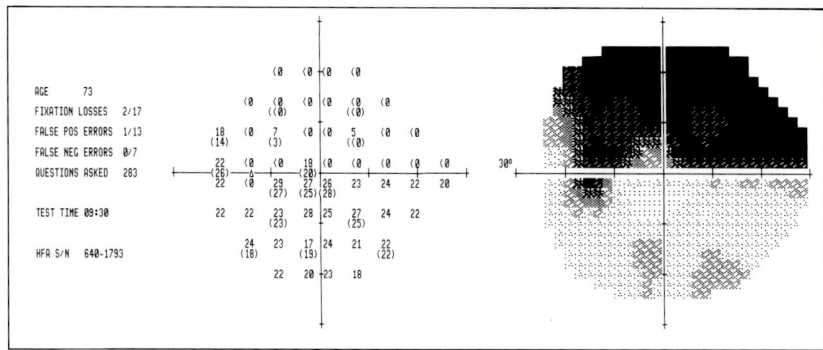

Figure B

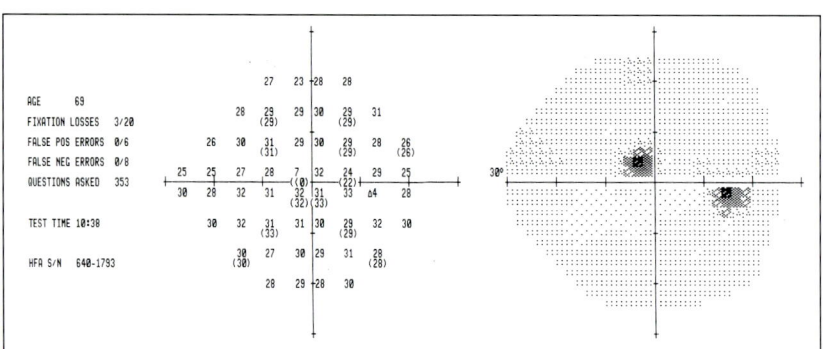

Figure C

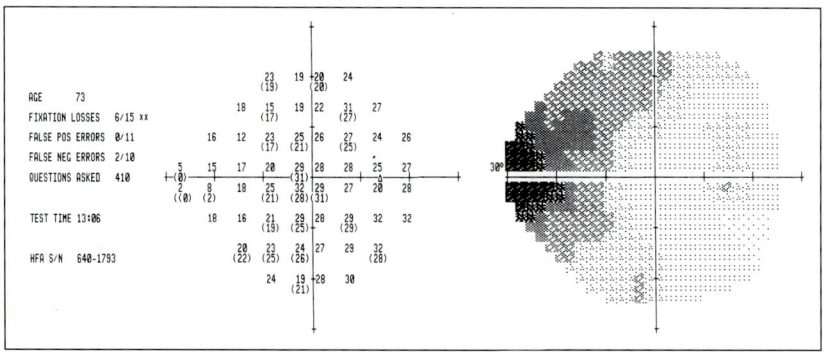

Figure D

a. Figure A
b. Figure B
c. Figure C
d. Figure D

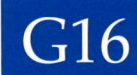

The figures below show typical glaucomatous optic nerve changes.

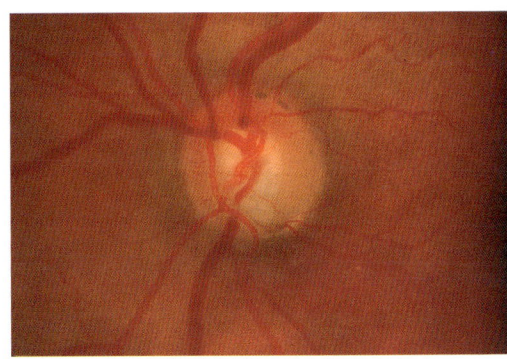

Figure A

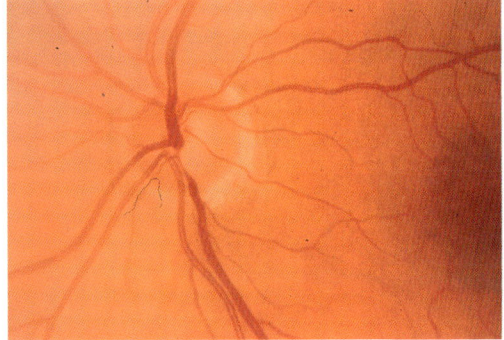

Figure B

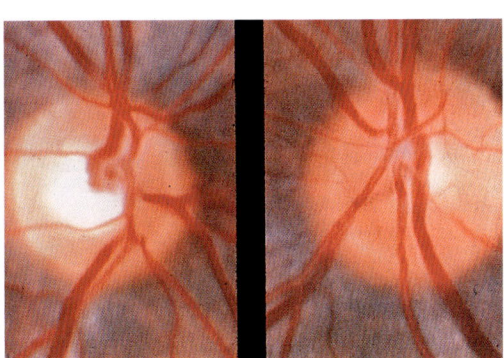

Figure C

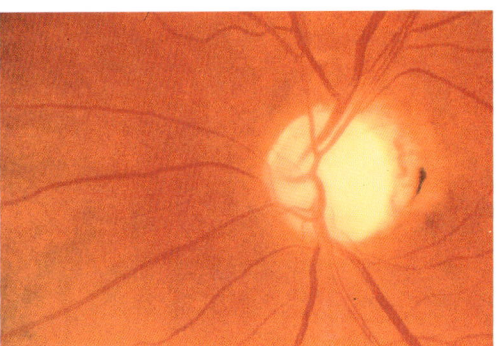

Figure D

Typical glaucomatous optic nerve changes can include all of the following *except*

a. notch in neuroretinal rim of the optic nerve (Figure A)
b. vertically oval optic cup (Figure B)
c. unilateral, asymmetric diffuse enlargement of optic disc cup (Figure C)
d. pallor of neuroretinal rim (pallor out of proportion to the degree of cupping) of optic nerve (Figure D)

G17 The problem requiring the *most* urgent management after glaucoma filtering surgery is

a. choroidal effusion
b. choroidal hemorrhage
c. shallow anterior chamber with iris-to-cornea touch
d. shallow anterior chamber with lens-to-cornea touch

G18 Laser trabeculoplasty is indicated for the management of uncontrolled glaucoma in all of the following situations *except*

a. active inflammatory (uveitic) glaucoma
b. exfoliation syndrome glaucoma
c. 35-year-old patient with pigmentary glaucoma
d. chronic primary angle-closure glaucoma with a patent laser iridotomy and one-third of angle closed by peripheral anterior synechiae

G19 All of the following are associated with chronic angle-closure glaucoma with relative pupillary block *except*

a. hyperopia
b. the presence of exfoliative material in the eye
c. cataract progression
d. peripheral radial iris transillumination defects

G20 All of the following will halt the progression of synechial angle closure in chronic primary angle-closure glaucoma *except*

a. cataract extraction
b. laser iridotomy
c. miotic (cholinergic) therapy
d. posterior lens dislocation

G21 A 66-year-old man had uncontrolled intraocular pressure on glaucoma medical therapy with a previous laser peripheral iridotomy for chronic angle closure. Five days after a trabeculectomy, he has a very shallow peripheral and central anterior chamber, patent iridotomy, intraocular pressure of 40 mm Hg, and no evidence of choroidal detachment on ocular B-scan ultrasonography. All of the following may help in the management of this patient *except*

a. miotic (cholinergic) therapy
b. topical beta blocker therapy
c. oral carbonic anhydrase inhibitor therapy
d. vitrectomy

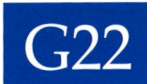
Exfoliation syndrome (pseudoexfoliation) glaucoma is associated with all of the following *except*

a. increased pigmentation of trabecular meshwork
b. zonular dehiscence
c. radial peripheral iris transillumination defects
d. chronic angle closure

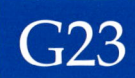
The *most* likely abnormality detected on automated perimetry in an ocular hypertensive patient with progressive nuclear sclerotic cataract would be

a. generalized depression, greater centrally
b. increased blind-spot size
c. depressed ring of peripheral points in a central 30° program
d. increased pattern standard deviation

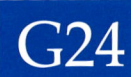
All of the following are reasons for an increased mean deviation on automated threshold perimetry *except*

a. cataract progression
b. glaucoma progression
c. high false-positive rate
d. topical miotic (cholinergic) therapy

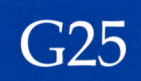
The *most* important finding suggestive of glaucoma in a patient with elevated intraocular pressure would be

a. cup-to-disc ratio asymmetry of 0.1
b. bilateral cup-to-disc ratio of 0.7
c. very deep optic cup
d. cup-to-disc ratio of 0.4 with notch formation in optic nerve rim

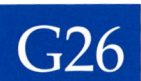
A 65-year-old man with severe proliferative diabetic retinopathy underwent a very heavy laser photocoagulation treatment session by your retinal associate 1 day previously. Today, the patient presents with mild pain, blurred vision, and an intraocular pressure of 45 mm Hg. Your retinal associate has already treated the patient with a topical beta blocker and oral carbonic anhydrase inhibitor and has referred him to you for further management of elevated intraocular pressure. The patient has no previous history of glaucoma and no evidence of iris neovascularization. On your examination, the anterior chamber appears very shallow and the fellow eye has a deep anterior chamber.

What would be the *most* appropriate initial management step?

a. Perform a laser iridotomy.
b. Perform a laser iridoplasty.
c. Give a topical cycloplegic agent.
d. Perform a trabeculectomy.

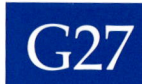
All of the following statements are true of the topical selective beta blocker betaxolol (Betoptic) *except*

a. It is less effective in lowering intraocular pressure than levobunolol (Betagan) or timolol (Timoptic).
b. It is safer for patients with mild, intermittent asthma attacks.
c. It has more additive effect of lowering intraocular pressure when combined with dipivefrin (Propine) than do the nonselective beta blockers.
d. It can be safely used in patients with congestive heart failure.

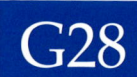
Laser iridotomy is indicated in all of the following *except*

a. neovascular glaucoma
b. chronic primary angle-closure glaucoma
c. pseudophakic pupillary-block glaucoma
d. inability to adequately view trabecular meshwork in an eye with narrow angle prior to performing laser trabeculoplasty

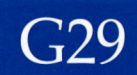
The *most* effective three-drug regimen for an eye with primary open-angle glaucoma would be

a. betaxolol, dipivefrin, pilocarpine
b. levobunolol, pilocarpine, acetazolamide
c. timolol, dipivefrin, carbachol
d. timolol, dipivefrin, acetazolamide

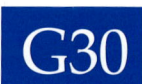
Two days after a trabeculectomy, a patient has an intraocular pressure of 3 mm Hg with a large bleb, no leak, and shallow but formed anterior chamber. On the third day, she presents stating that she developed moderate pain and decreased vision after bending over. The visual acuity is finger-counting and the intraocular pressure is 37 mm Hg. The bleb is unchanged in appearance. There is a moderate-sized, dark, temporal choroidal detachment. The lens and vitreous are clear, and there is no evidence of a retinal detachment.

All of the following are appropriate actions at this time *except*

a. perform drainage of choroidal hemorrhage
b. add topical beta blocker to reduce intraocular pressure
c. continue topical corticosteroid therapy
d. add cycloplegic therapy

G31 A 78-year-old man experienced unilateral sudden loss of vision 1 year previously. Currently, he complains of severe pain in that eye. Examination reveals no light-perception vision, intraocular pressure of 72 mm Hg, iris neovascularization, and evidence of a central retinal vein occlusion.

The *least* helpful therapeutic agent at this time would be

a. topical cycloplegic
b. topical corticosteroid
c. topical beta blocker
d. topical cholinergic (miotic) agent

G32 Which of the following statements is true of apraclonidine (Iopidine)?

a. It is an alpha-1 adrenergic agonist.
b. It commonly causes systemic hypotension.
c. It may cause transient lid retraction.
d. It is associated with macular edema in aphakic eyes.

G33 A 21-year-old woman with juvenile open-angle glaucoma and 7 diopters of myopia complains of severe blurring of vision after using 1 drop of pilocarpine. The *most* likely cause of her symptom is

a. a small pupil
b. increased hyperopia
c. increased myopia
d. retinal detachment

G34 Two years after a successful filtering procedure (full-thickness sclerectomy), a patient complains of pain, tearing, and blurred vision for 2 days. The visual acuity is 20/50, the intraocular pressure is 4 mm Hg, the bleb is flat, and there is a rare cell in the anterior chamber.

The *most* likely explanation of these symptoms and signs is

a. endophthalmitis
b. retinal detachment
c. bleb leak
d. ciliary body detachment

G35 All of the following statements about chronic primary angle-closure glaucoma are true *except*

a. It can develop in a patient with primary open-angle glaucoma.
b. It can develop in a myopic eye.
c. It often causes no pain.
d. It can be prevented by pilocarpine therapy.

G36 A miotic agent would be *least* effective in a patient with glaucoma and which one of the following?

a. aniridia with open angle
b. angle recession
c. aphakia
d. severe secondary angle closure

G37 Glaucoma-like visual field defects can be seen in all of the following conditions *except*

a. cerebrovascular accident
b. buried optic nerve drusen
c. retinal vascular occlusion
d. ischemic optic neuropathy

G38 A patient with elevated intraocular pressure undergoes automated static threshold perimetry. Most threshold determinations are high (40 dB to 50 dB). What is the *most* likely reason for this?

a. alert but nervous patient
b. drowsy patient
c. media opacity
d. end-stage glaucoma

G39 Lens extraction may resolve glaucoma in all of the following situations *except*

a. microspherophakia
b. phacolytic glaucoma
c. exfoliation syndrome (pseudoexfoliation) glaucoma
d. chronic primary angle-closure glaucoma

G40 Which of the following statements is true about corticosteroid-induced intraocular pressure elevation?

a. It usually begins within 1 day after beginning corticosteroid therapy.
b. It is more common in patients with primary open-angle glaucoma than in patients with ocular hypertension.
c. Intraocular pressure usually does not return to baseline levels after discontinuing the corticosteroid.
d. Fluorinated corticosteroids usually cause a greater incidence of intraocular pressure elevation than nonfluorinated corticosteroid preparations.

G41 Which of the following is the *most* helpful clue in the diagnosis of chronic primary angle-closure glaucoma?

a. amount of glaucomatous optic nerve damage at presentation
b. gonioscopic findings
c. level of intraocular pressure at presentation
d. ocular symptoms (pain, haloes)

G42 A 58-year-old man presents to your office with a history of primary open-angle glaucoma and intraocular pressures of 20 mm Hg OU using a topical beta blocker twice daily and pilocarpine 4%, 3 times daily to both eyes. Gonioscopy reveals open angles and light trabecular pigmentation. You dilate the patient's pupils with two sets of tropicamide 1% and phenylephrine 2.5% drops in each eye. One hour later, you return to perform the dilated examination and the patient complains of blurred vision. There is mild corneal edema, and the intraocular pressure is 44 mm Hg bilaterally.

Which of the following is the *most* likely reason for this acute elevation of intraocular pressure?

a. idiosyncratic reaction to one of the dilating agents
b. hypersensitivity to one of the dilating agents
c. angle closure
d. reversal of intraocular pressure–lowering effect of glaucoma medication by one of the dilating agents

G43 Topical ocular beta blockers have been reported to cause all of the following side effects *except*

a. heart block
b. exacerbation of myasthenia gravis
c. hypokalemia
d. blockage of the systemic response to hypoglycemia in diabetic patients

G44 Topical ocular beta blockers could have a beneficial effect on all of the following disorders *except*

a. supraventricular tachyarrhythmia
b. systemic hypertension
c. second-degree heart block
d. angina pectoris

G45 All of the following statements are true about dipivefrin (Propine) *except*

a. It is more lipophilic than topical ocular epinephrine formulations.
b. Systemic effects are equally likely with dipivefrin and epinephrine.
c. It is formulated in a lower concentration than the epinephrine formulations.
d. It is more likely to cause contact dermatitis than a topical ocular beta adrenergic antagonist.

G46 During a trabeculectomy, the block excision is performed 1 mm to 2 mm too far posteriorly. Possible complications of this may include all of the following *except*

a. inadvertent cyclodialysis cleft
b. hemorrhage
c. focal corneal edema
d. vitreous loss

G47 A 2-year-old child presents with bilateral findings shown in the figures.

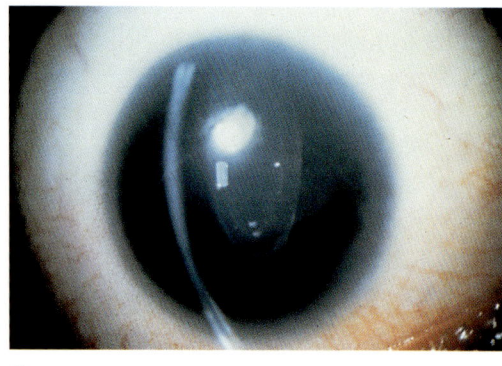

A

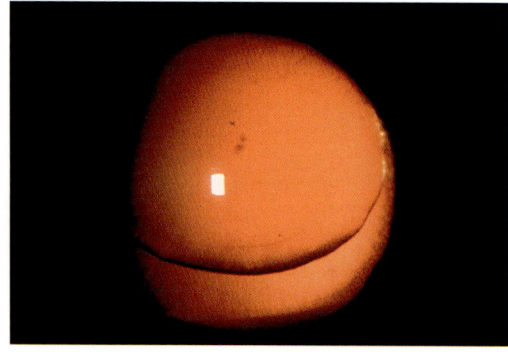

B

Possible findings would include all of the following *except*

a. peripheral corneal pannus
b. neuroblastoma (Wilms' tumor)
c. angle-closure glaucoma
d. adhesions of peripheral iris to a prominent, anteriorly displaced Schwalbe's line

G48 Observe the optic nerve in the photograph below.

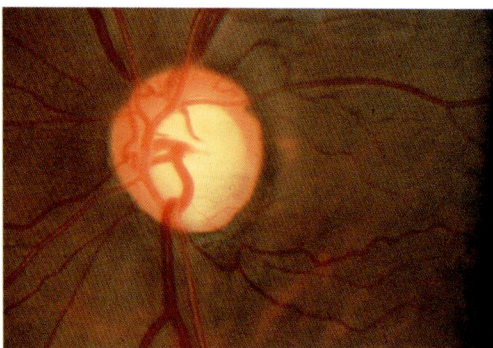

Which of the four visual field tests would best match this optic nerve?

SECTION ONE: GLAUCOMA

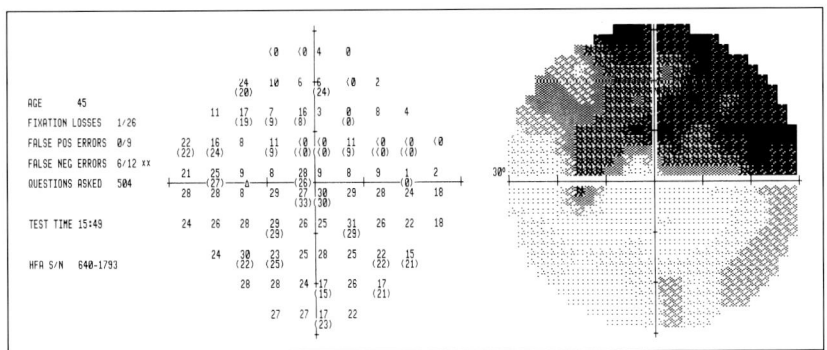

Figure A

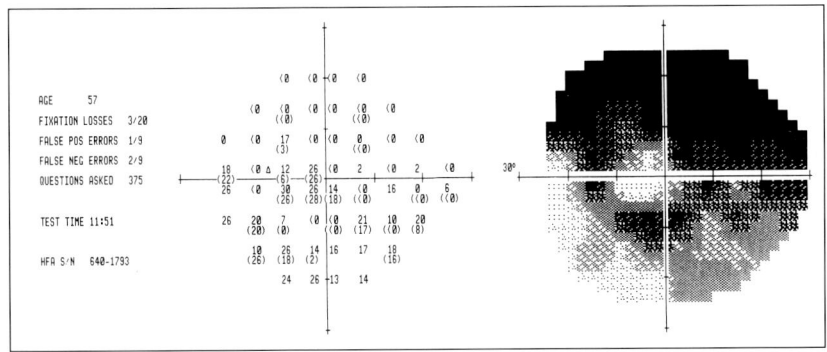

Figure B

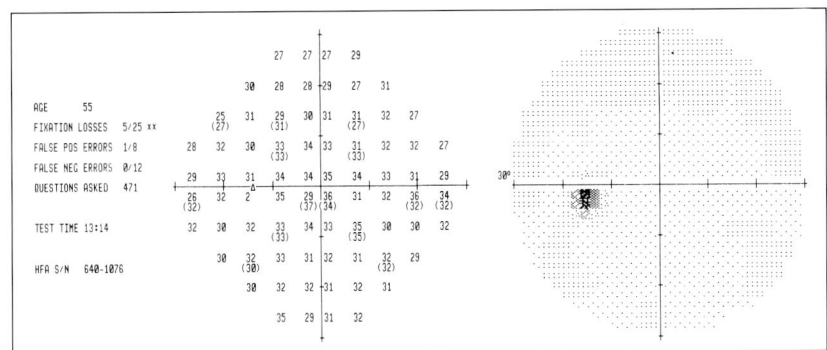

Figure C

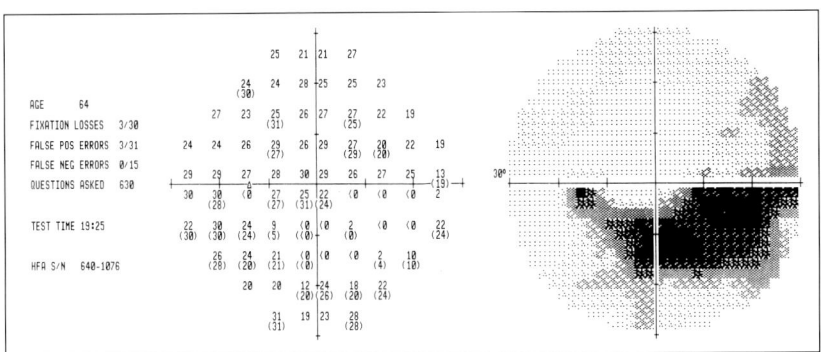

Figure D

a. Figure A
b. Figure B
c. Figure C
d. Figure D

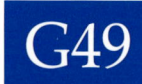
A 35-year-old woman presents with the clinical findings in the right eye shown in the figures. The intraocular pressure is 38 mm Hg, and gonioscopy shows extensive peripheral anterior synechiae in that eye.

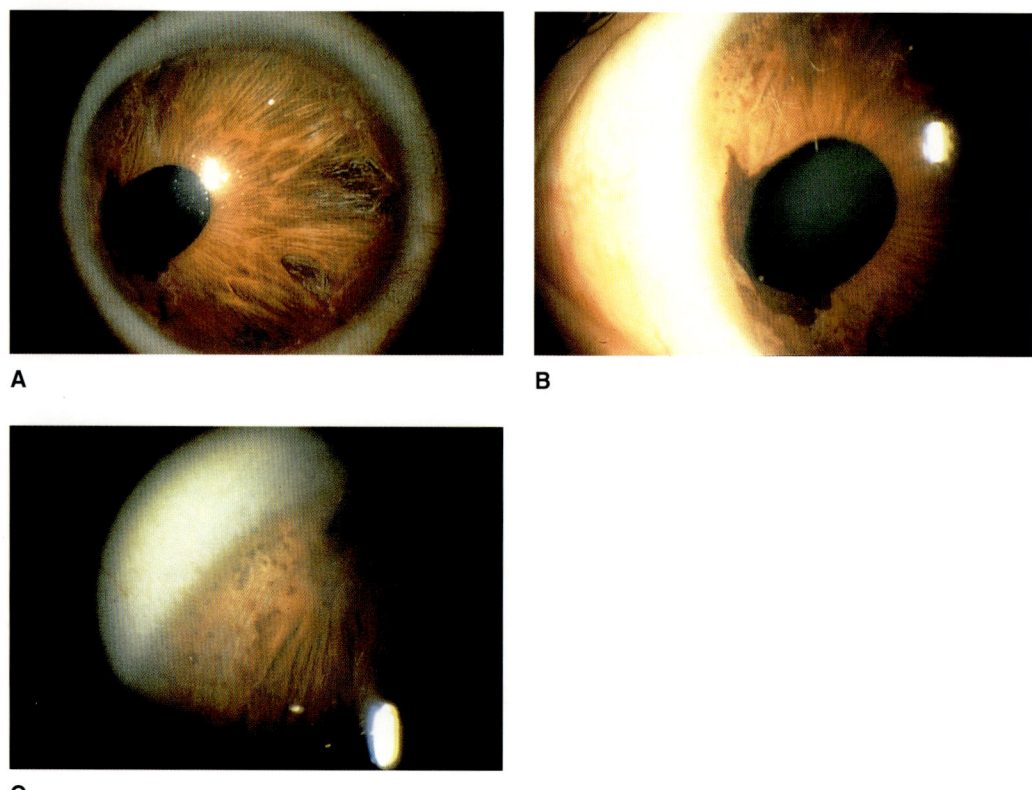

Which one of the following is *most* likely to provide the greatest reduction of intraocular pressure?

- a. acetazolamide
- b. laser iridotomy
- c. laser trabeculoplasty
- d. topical corticosteroid

SECTION ONE: GLAUCOMA

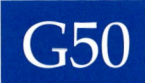

Which of the gonioscopic photographs shown below would represent a normal anatomic finding?

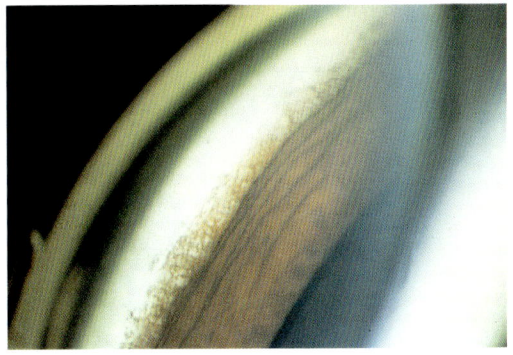

Figure A

Figure B

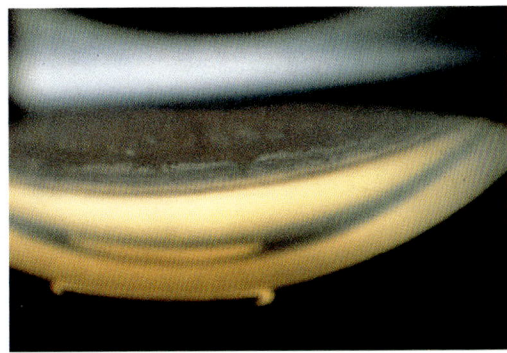

Figure C

Figure D

a. Figure A
b. Figure B
c. Figure C
d. Figure D

SECTION TWO
EXTERNAL DISEASE AND CORNEA

E1 A 6-year-old boy has developed a pink mass on the inside of the lower lid that has enlarged rapidly (see the figure). The mass is associated with marked mucus production.

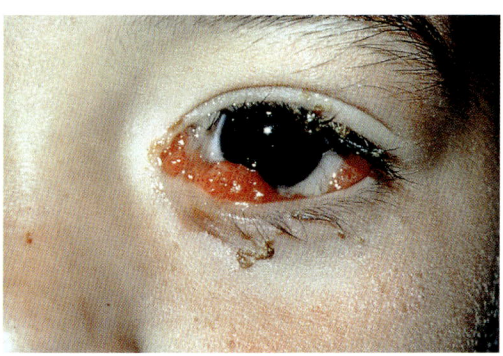

The *most* likely diagnosis is

a. squamous cell carcinoma
b. rhabdomyosarcoma
c. conjunctival papilloma
d. lymphogranuloma venereum

E2 The *most* likely cause of the lesion in the patient in Question E1 is

a. actinic trauma
b. viral infection
c. herpes simplex
d. *Chlamydia psittaci*

E3 All of the following features are characteristic of the condition diagnosed in the patient in Question E1 *except*

a. tendency to recur and spread to other sites on the ocular surface after excision
b. predilection for the conjunctival fornix
c. frequent malignant degeneration
d. occurrence at multiple sites in a single eye

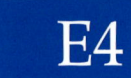

A 57-year-old farmer is referred to the ophthalmologist by a family practitioner for management of chronic conjunctivitis that has been unresponsive to topical antibiotics or antibiotic/corticosteroid combinations for more than 10 weeks. The patient has a painless red eye that produces a mucoserous discharge. His ocular lesion is shown in the figure.

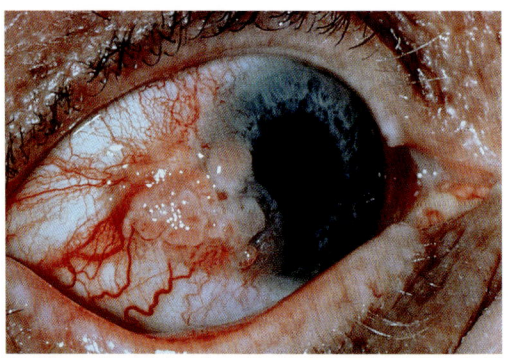

The *most* likely diagnosis is

a. squamous cell carcinoma of the conjunctiva
b. ocular pemphigoid
c. drug toxicity
d. acanthosis nigricans

Lesions of the type shown in the figure in Question E4 tend to have all of the following characteristics *except*

a. They are most commonly unifocal.
b. They tend to be slow growing.
c. They are generally exophytic.
d. They invade the intraocular space 50% of the time.

The figure shows a corneal lesion with a fimbriated border pattern.

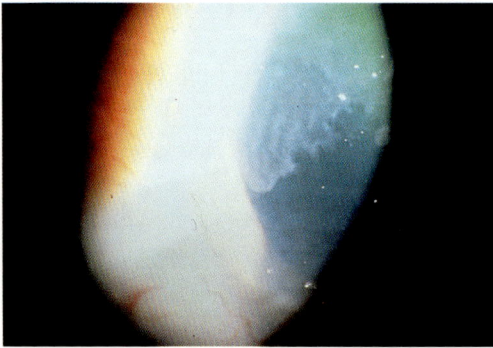

This lesion is *most* likely to be

a. squamous dysplasia
b. corneal nevus
c. fibrous outgrowth
d. leukoplakia

E7 The *most* appropriate surgical management of squamous cell carcinoma of the conjunctiva is

a. wide marginal conjunctivectomy with deep anterior sclerectomy
b. beta-irradiation
c. superficial excision with adjuvant cryoablation
d. cryoablation alone

E8 A 25-year-old Hispanic woman has noticed a change in a brown spot on her right eye. Although she states that the spot has been present since she was 14 years old, she and her family have noticed a distinct enlargement and deepening of the pigment over the last 4 months (see the figure). She is concerned that the lesion may represent a developing cancer. Aside from the lesion, her external examination is unremarkable.

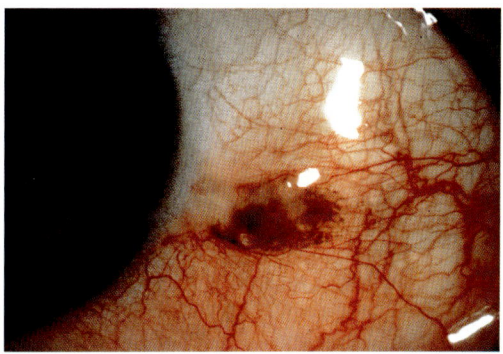

The *most* likely diagnosis of the lesion is

a. nevus of Ota
b. malignant melanoma of the conjunctiva
c. benign conjunctival nevus
d. squamous cell carcinoma

E9 Initial management of the lesion in Question E8 might include all of the following *except*

a. baseline photographic documentation
b. excisional biopsy
c. review of old facial photographs
d. cryoablation

E10 A 38-year-old blond woman who works as a forest ranger reports first noting the appearance of a brown lesion on the right eye 4 months ago. Since then the lesion has grown in size and darkened in pigmentation (see the figures). She denies any inflammation or ocular discomfort.

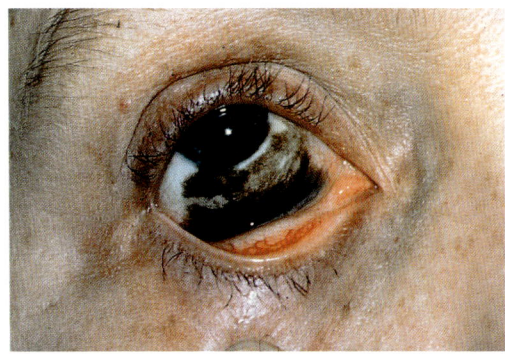
A

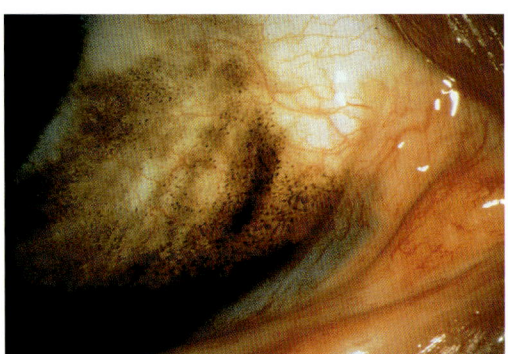
B

The *most* likely diagnosis of this lesion is

a. congenital melanosis of the conjunctiva
b. primary acquired melanosis
c. benign nevus
d. ochronosis

E11 The patient described in Question E10 has been advised by her grandmother, who is being treated for glaucoma, that these lesions run in the family, as evidenced by the pigmented lesions she has had in her own eye (shown below) for several years.

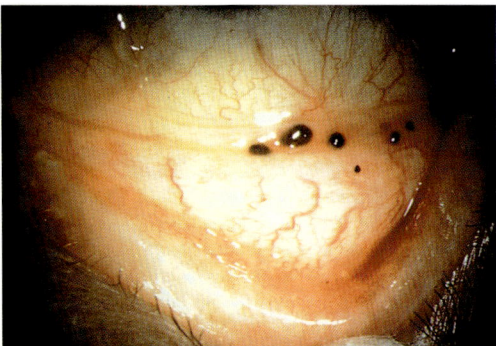

These lesions in the grandmother *most* likely represent

a. conjunctival nevi
b. malignant melanoma
c. adrenochrome deposits
d. congenital melanosis

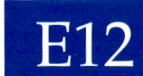 The patient in Question E10 returned 1 month later with a palpable mass in the upper lid. Eversion of the upper lid revealed the deeply pigmented mass pictured below.

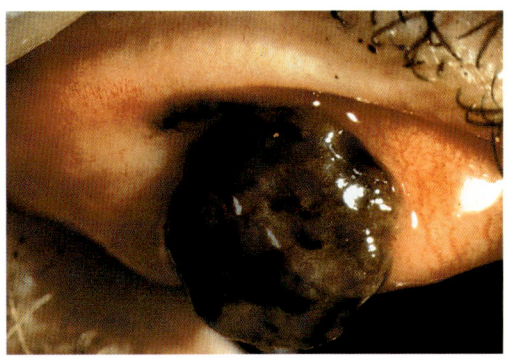

The *most* likely diagnosis is

a. adrenochrome deposit
b. pyogenic granuloma
c. acanthosis nigricans
d. malignant melanoma

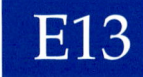 The appropriate management of malignant melanoma of the conjunctiva is

a. observation only, since there is a negligible mortality rate from these tumors
b. excision with adjunct cryoablation of raised pigmented lesions
c. PUVA (psoralens plus ultraviolet A) therapy
d. beta-irradiation

E14 A college basketball player who wears extended-wear soft contact lenses presents at the ophthalmologist's office after 2 days of pain, redness, and photophobia. He noticed an enlarging spot on his cornea (see the figure) 24 hours prior to coming to the doctor's office.

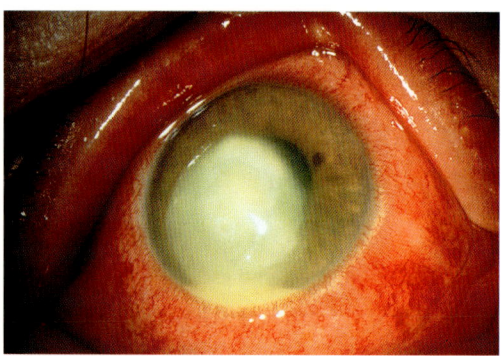

The *most* appropriate initial step in managing this problem is

a. immediate treatment with a single broad-spectrum topical antibiotic
b. subconjunctival injection of antibiotics
c. diagnostic scrapings of the corneal lesion for Gram stain and culture
d. treatment with an antibiotic/corticosteroid combination

E15 The patient in Question E14 is initially managed on the basis of the results of the Gram stain performed in the ophthalmologist's office (see the figure).

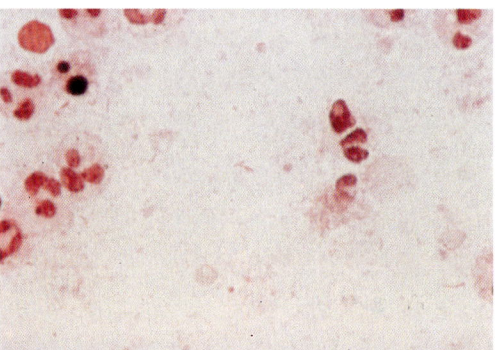

The findings are *most* consistent with

a. *Pseudomonas aeruginosa*
b. *Neisseria gonorrhoeae*
c. *Streptococcus pneumoniae*
d. *Staphylococcus aureus*

E16 A thorough discussion of the history of the contact lens habits of the patient in Question E14 revealed that he wore the lenses 24 hours a day and removed them for cleaning every 2 weeks. At the time of removal, he used chemical disinfection and then, to ensure sterility, stored the lenses in distilled water overnight prior to reinsertion. He noted that he did not routinely clean his storage apparatus.

All of these historical points are significant for the development of contact-lens–related infection *except*

a. 24-hour wear
b. use of distilled water for sterility
c. failure to maintain clean storage apparatus
d. chemical disinfection

E17 A 62-year-old woman has been followed for corneal decompensation from Fuchs' dystrophy. She has demonstrated gradual progression from asymptomatic cornea guttata to stromal edema and frank bullous keratopathy over 4 years. She now complains of severe pain, photophobia, and tearing that has lasted for 5 days. Her cornea appears as shown in the figure.

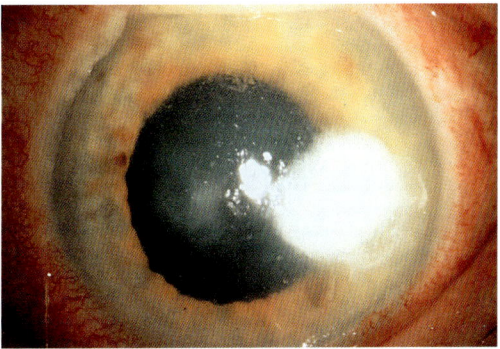

The findings are *most* consistent with

a. painful bullous keratopathy
b. secondary bacterial keratitis
c. herpes simplex keratitis
d. *Acanthamoeba* keratitis

E18 The patient in Question E17 is diagnosed with staphylococcal keratitis, established by Gram stain and bacterial cultures. The antibiotic of choice for initial therapy would *most* likely be from which class of drugs?

a. macrolides (eg, erythromycin)
b. cephalosporins (eg, cefazolin)
c. imidazoles (eg, miconazole)
d. fluoroquinolones (eg, ciprofloxacin)

E19 In examining the patient in Question E17, the treating ophthalmologist notes the presence of a hypopyon in association with the corneal infiltrate. The hypopyon

a. indicates that there is a concomitant endophthalmitis and calls for an anterior chamber tap
b. is invariably present with bacterial keratitis
c. is a reactive inflammatory response and does not necessarily indicate intraocular infection
d. is more likely to occur with *Acanthamoeba* than with staphylococcal infection

E20 A 57-year-old man complains of redness, intense foreign-body sensation, and photophobia that has lasted for 1 week. He states that he has had these episodes several times before. As shown in the figure, there are several small, white infiltrates near the inferior limbus with overlying epithelial defects. Examination of the patient reveals, in addition, the presence of significant lid inflammation.

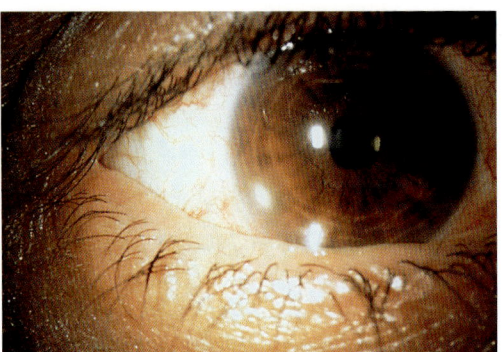

The *most* likely diagnosis would be

a. *Pseudomonas* keratitis
b. herpes simplex keratitis
c. staphylococcal marginal keratitis
d. Terrien's marginal degeneration

E21 The management of the disorder diagnosed in the patient in Question E20 includes all of the following *except*

a. topical corticosteroids
b. lid hygiene
c. topical antibiotic
d. prophylactic antiviral drops

E22 A debilitated 63-year-old man who lives on the streets had developed a red, painful eye 5 days prior to seeing an ophthalmologist. His cornea at the time of examination is shown in the figure, part A. The results of Gram staining of corneal scrapings are shown in part B of the figure.

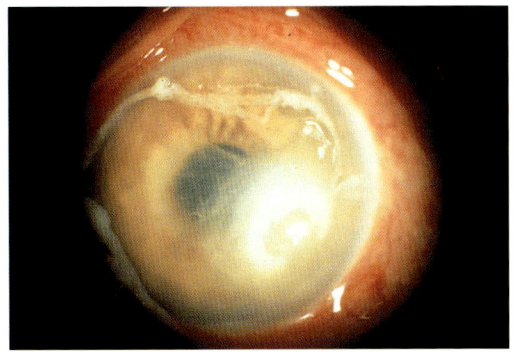
A

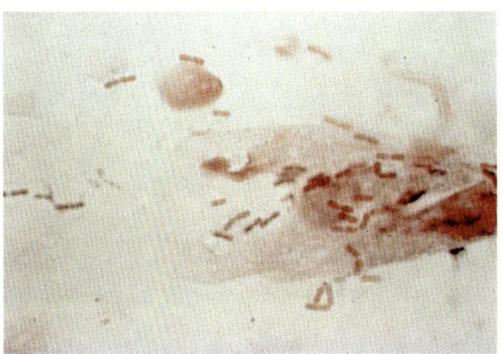
B

The organism *most* likely involved is

a. *Pseudomonas aeruginosa*
b. *Klebsiella pneumoniae*
c. *Moraxella lacunata*
d. *Neisseria gonorrhoeae*

E23 A 47-year-old electrician was working under a house when some dirt was dislodged from a beam overhead and fell into his eye. He flushed out the eye on the site and went about his work. Two days later, he developed a red, painful eye and mild photophobia. Symptoms became progressively worse over the next week. He was seen by a family practitioner, who gave him an eyedrop containing antibiotic and corticosteroid. He then noticed a white spot in the center of his cornea while shaving and saw the ophthalmologist. The lesion in the photograph did not stain with fluorescein.

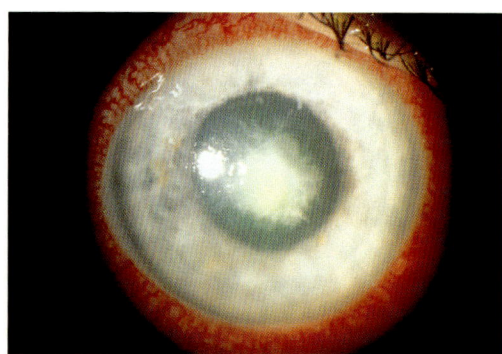

The history and appearance of the lesion are *most* consistent with

a. fungal keratitis
b. *Acanthamoeba* keratitis
c. herpes simplex keratitis
d. Gram-negative ulcer

E24 The appropriate laboratory workup of the ulcer presented in Question E23 would include all of the following measures *except*

a. scraping for Giemsa stain
b. plating on Sabouraud's agar
c. plating on blood agar to be maintained at room temperature
d. plating on nonnutrient agar with a lawn of *E coli*

E25 The patient in Question E23 developed fungal cultures positive for *Aspergillus.* Based on the initial laboratory workup and later on the cultures, he was treated with an antimicrobial. All of the following classes of drugs might be considered *except*

a. imidazoles (eg, miconazole and ketoconazole)
b. polyenes (eg, amphotericin B and natamycin)
c. macrolides (eg, tetracycline and erythromycin)
d. pyrimidines (eg, flucytosine)

E26 Despite aggressive therapy with antifungal agents, the lesion of the patient in Question E23 progressed and began to melt centrally. Medications were stopped and the cornea was scraped and recultured. Once again, hyphal elements were seen and *Aspergillus* grew on agar plates. At this point the *most* reasonable therapeutic option would be

a. therapeutic penetrating keratoplasty
b. lamellar keratoplasty
c. treatment with propamidine isethionate
d. chemical cautery

E27 A 32-year-old Caucasian man complains to the ophthalmologist of bilateral intermittent redness, lacrimation, and foreign-body sensation. The most recent episode has been associated with extreme, almost disabling, photophobia. His lesion is shown in the figure.

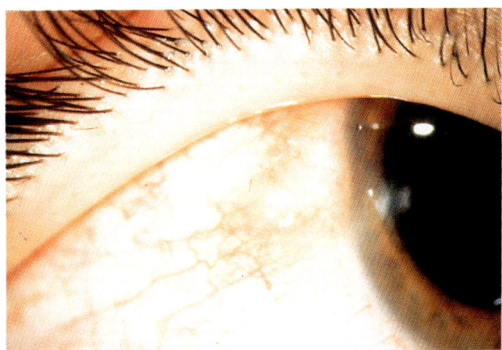

This lesion is *most* consistent with

a. superior limbic keratoconjunctivitis
b. phlyctenulosis
c. Thygeson's superficial punctate keratitis
d. staphylococcal marginal keratitis

E28 The most common cause of the condition diagnosed in Question E27 is

a. tuberculosis
b. *Staphylococcus aureus*
c. *Moraxella* infection
d. *Streptococcus pneumoniae*

E29 A 73-year-old man presents to the ophthalmologist with a 10-day history of accelerating discomfort and red eye. The patient exhibits signs of intense pain. Examination reveals a sharply demarcated peripheral corneal ulceration with a central overhanging edge (see the figure).

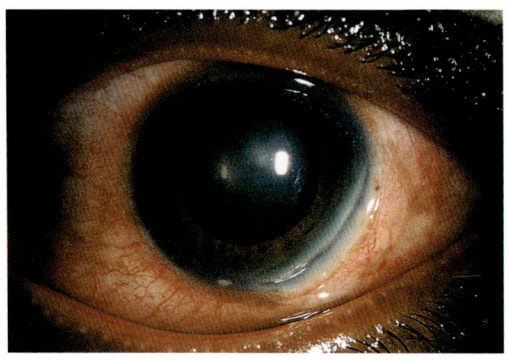

The *most* likely diagnosis is

a. Terrien's marginal degeneration
b. staphylococcal marginal keratitis
c. senile marginal furrow
d. Mooren's ulcer

E30 Therapeutic approaches for the ulcer shown in Question E29 include all of the following *except*

a. topical corticosteroids
b. systemic immunosuppressive agents
c. conjunctival resection
d. topical nonsteroidal anti-inflammatory agents

E31 A 66-year-old woman presents with redness, pain, and decreased vision in the left eye that has lasted for 2 weeks. She is noted to have an area of ulceration and extreme thinning at the limbus (see the figure, part A), and, in addition, she has a moderately dry eye. Her hands appear as shown in part B of the figure.

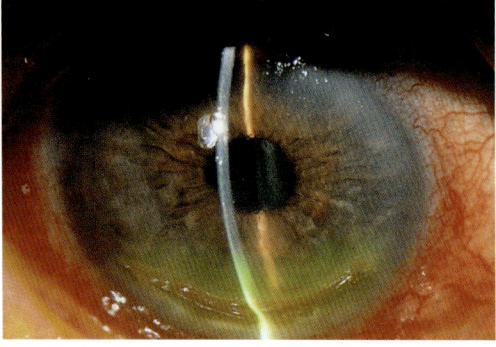
A

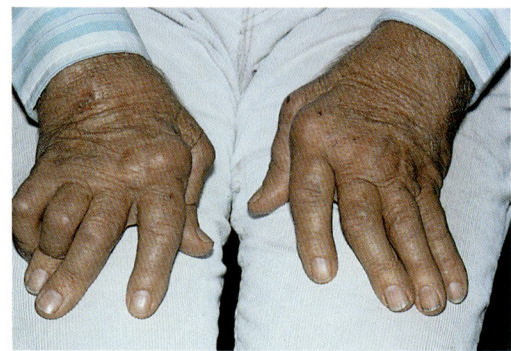
B

The *most* likely diagnosis in this case is

a. rheumatoid marginal corneal ulceration
b. Mooren's ulcer
c. Terrien's marginal degeneration
d. sclerokeratitis

E32 All of the following treatments are appropriate for the management of the problem of the patient in Question E31 *except*

a. conjunctival resection
b. topical corticosteroids
c. topical collagenase inhibitors
d. lamellar keratoplasty

E33 A 43-year-old woman presents with irritation and a gritty sensation in both eyes. These symptoms have been present for several months but have worsened during the dry summer season and tend to worsen as the day goes on. She is otherwise in good health. The figure shows the result of fluorescein staining.

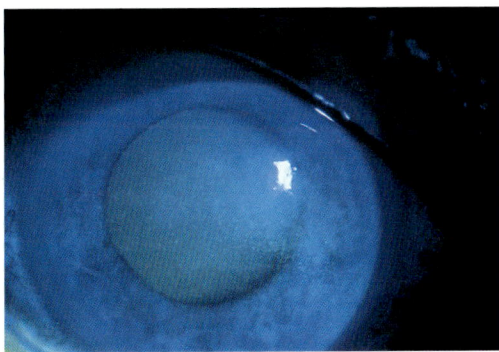

All of the following abnormalities in a patient with aqueous-deficiency dry eye might be expected *except*

a. decreased tear meniscus
b. abnormal Schirmer test
c. diminished tear break-up time
d. increased mucus in the precorneal tear film and/or filamentary keratitis

E34 Appropriate therapy of keratitis sicca includes all of the following *except*

a. application of mucolytic agents
b. punctal occlusion
c. topical corticosteroids
d. tear substitutes

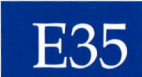 A 26-year-old woman who wears rigid gas-permeable lenses 14 to 16 hours a day complains of a scratchy sensation after 6 to 8 hours of wearing time. Examination of the corneal surface reveals the staining pattern shown in the figure.

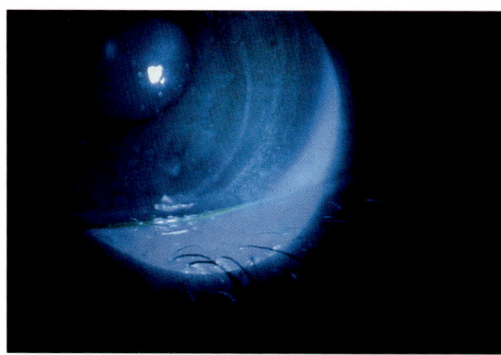

All of the following statements about this condition are true *except*

a. It is referred to as 3 and 9 o'clock staining.
b. It may result from peripheral desiccation of the cornea.
c. It is uncommon in wearers of gas-permeable contact lenses.
d. It can be managed by lubrication, alterations in lens design, or conversion to hydrogel lenses.

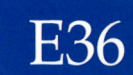 A 34-year-old man visits the ophthalmologist 3 weeks after being fit with new rigid gas-permeable contact lenses. He complains of hazy vision, particularly after removing the lenses and using his glasses. Examination of the cornea reveals the findings shown in the figure.

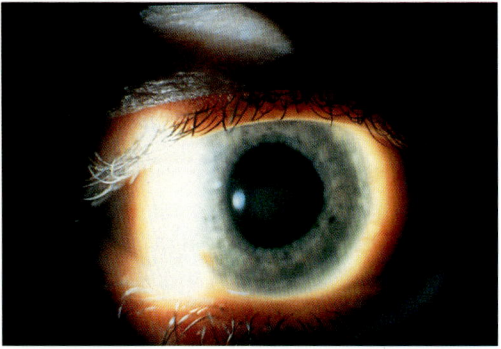

The cause of this problem is

a. a lens that is too loosely fit
b. hypersensitivity to proteins on the lens surface
c. epithelial hypoxia
d. stromal edema

E37 A 67-year-old woman complains of foreign-body sensation, tearing, and photophobia in her left eye, in which the vision has been poor for several years. The figure shows the result of biomicroscopic examination.

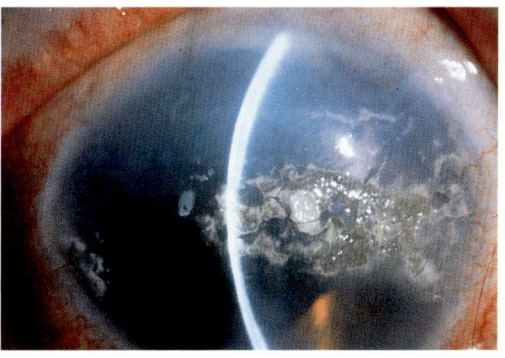

The *most* likely diagnosis is

a. calcific band keratopathy
b. Salzmann's nodular degeneration
c. central cloudy cornea of François
d. spheroid degeneration

E38 Management of the condition diagnosed in the patient in Question E37 includes all of the following *except*

a. bandage contact lens
b. chelation with disodium EDTA
c. application of silver nitrate
d. scraping

E39 A 12-year-old boy underwent penetrating keratoplasty for complications of herpes simplex keratitis. He was managed with a routine regimen of prednisolone acetate and a prophylactic regimen of topical antiviral medication for the first several weeks. His postoperative course was uncomplicated until he developed an area of focal injection near a graft suture and an adjacent superficial anterior stromal crystalline deposit in the clear cornea (see the figure).

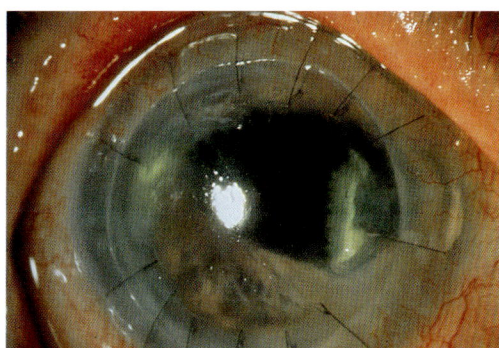

The *most* likely diagnosis is

a. recurrent herpes simplex keratitis
b. bacterial keratitis
c. fungal keratitis
d. steroid crystallization

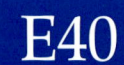

The *least* appropriate antibiotic for the management of the condition of the patient in Question E39 is

a. vancomycin
b. cefazolin
c. gentamicin
d. penicillin

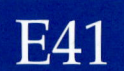

All of the following may produce crystalline deposits in the cornea *except*

a. systemic paraproteinemias
b. cystinosis
c. chlorpromazine
d. streptococcal infection

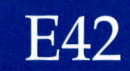

A 19-year-old college student complains of poor vision. He states that he has long been nearsighted but that his glasses have recently required several changes, and even with his most recent correction, he is having difficulty. Examination reveals a best-corrected acuity of 20/40 with spectacle correction. The results of slit-lamp biomicroscopy are shown in the figures.

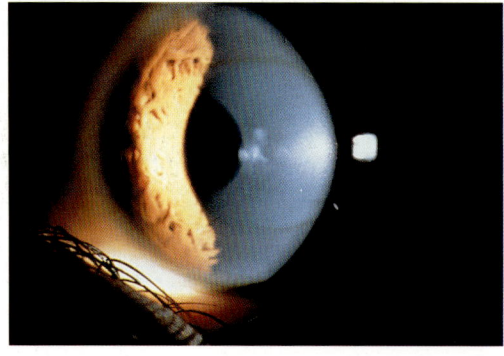
A

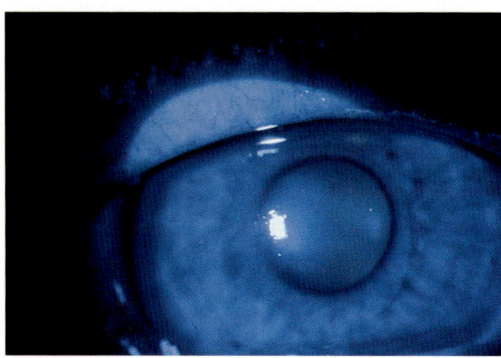
B

The *most* likely diagnosis is

a. keratoconus
b. pellucid marginal degeneration
c. Terrien's marginal degeneration
d. keratoglobus

SECTION TWO: EXTERNAL DISEASE AND CORNEA

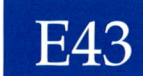

E43 Other findings associated with the condition found in the patient in Question E42 include all of the following *except*

a. pre-Descemet's striae
b. apical reticular scarring and thinning
c. peripheral vascularization
d. inferior corneal steepening

E44 Of the computer-assisted topographic analyses shown below, which is *most* likely to correspond with the patient in Question E42?

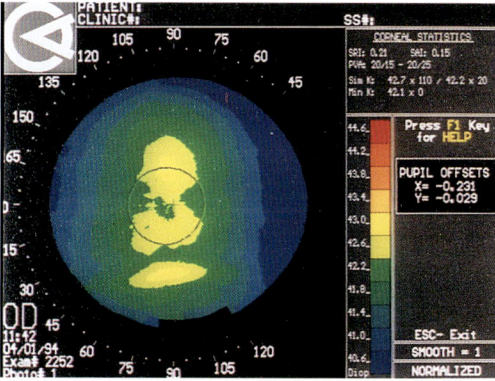

Figure A

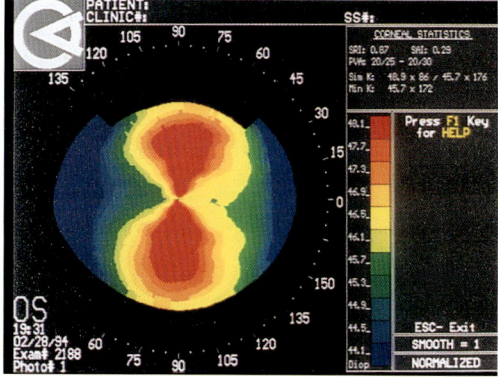

Figure B

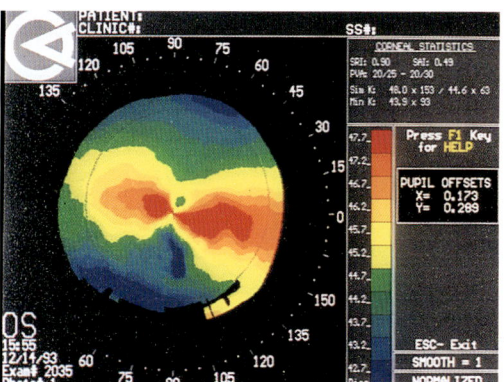

Figure C

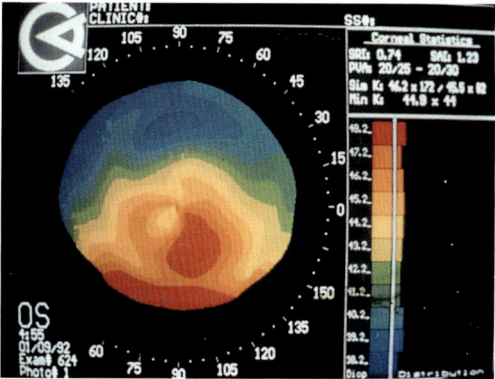

Figure D

a. Figure A
b. Figure B
c. Figure C
d. Figure D

E45

A patient with keratoconus is fit with a rigid gas-permeable contact lens. The patient's fluorescein pattern is shown below.

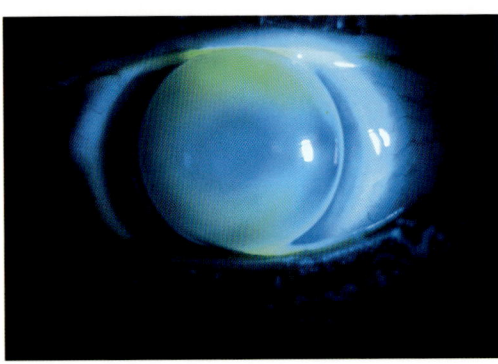

Which of the following characteristics does the fluorescein pattern demonstrate?

a. central bearing
b. peripheral touch
c. a lens that is too steep
d. tight lens syndrome

E46

The lens–cornea relationship in the patient in Question E45 is the best achievable fit leading to stability of position and acceptable vision. The *most* appropriate measure at this point in the patient's management is to

a. abandon contact lens fitting and suggest keratoplasty
b. let the patient try the lens
c. consider a central flattening procedure to facilitate lens fit
d. perform radial keratotomy

E47

The patient in Question E45 is happy with the fit of his contact lenses. However, 6 months later, he calls the office and agitatedly explains that he saw his family practitioner for a red eye that he developed 3 days ago. The family doctor told him that he had a serious corneal infection, prescribed antibiotics, and referred him to you for treatment. The lesion appears as shown in the figure. There is no epithelial defect, and the anterior chamber is deep and has only slight flare and a few cells. However, you note photophobia, tearing, conjunctival hyperemia, and vision decreased to bare finger-counting.

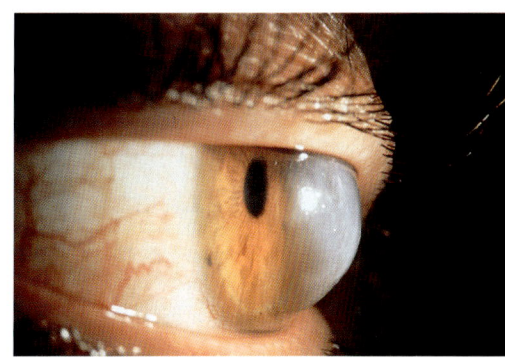

The *most* likely diagnosis is

a. bacterial keratitis
b. *Acanthamoeba* keratitis
c. acute corneal hydrops
d. corneal perforation

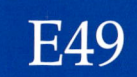 The *most* appropriate management of the problem in Question E47 is

a. keratoplasty
b. cyclopentolate and topical hypertonic salt solution
c. therapeutic contact lens
d. antibiotics

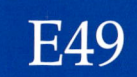 A 65-year-old woman complains of deep, boring pain of 3 days' duration. She denies any visual deficits, but she is unable to sleep because of the accelerating pain. Her eye is shown in the figure.

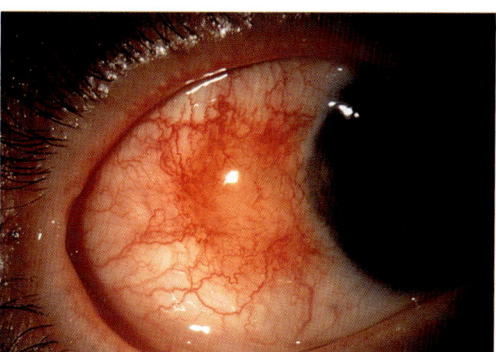

The clinical picture is *most* consistent with

a. interstitial keratitis
b. nodular scleritis
c. conjunctivitis
d. anterior uveitis

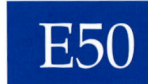

All of the following laboratory tests would be appropriate in the workup of the patient in Question E49 *except*

a. serum glucose
b. fluorescent treponemal antibody absorption (FTA-ABS)
c. antinuclear antibody (ANA)
d. rheumatoid factor (RF)

SECTION THREE
Cataract and Anterior Segment Surgery

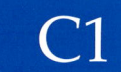

A patient is noted to have the cataract shown in the slit-lamp photograph below.

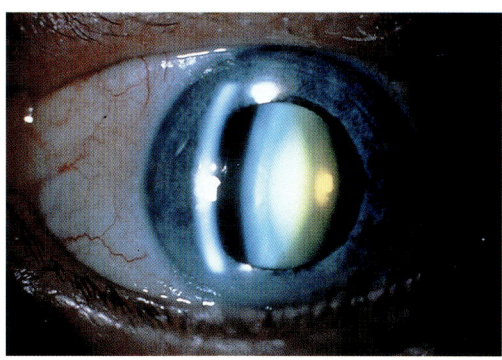

Cataracts of this type may be associated with all of the following *except*

a. early loss of near (reading) vision
b. a myopic shift
c. monocular diplopia
d. difficulty seeing road signs at dusk

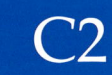

On pupillary dilation, a patient shows the characteristic lens change shown in the figure.

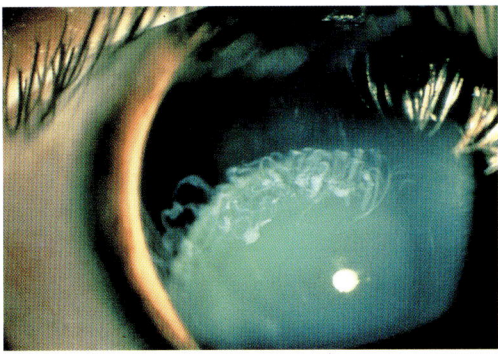

The *least* likely diagnosis is

a. Marfan syndrome
b. homocystinuria
c. Weill-Marchesani syndrome
d. Sturge-Weber syndrome

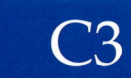 An 80-year-old woman underwent uneventful phacoemulsification and polymethylmethacrylate (PMMA) IOL implantation. She was noted to have an axial length of 21.8 mm and exfoliation syndrome with a maximally dilated pupil of 5.5 mm preoperatively. A 4.5 mm capsulorhexis was performed at surgery and a 5.5 mm optic, 12 mm overall length IOL was placed within the capsular bag. Three weeks after surgery, a contraction of the capsulorhexis opening to approximately 3.5 mm is noted, as shown in the figure.

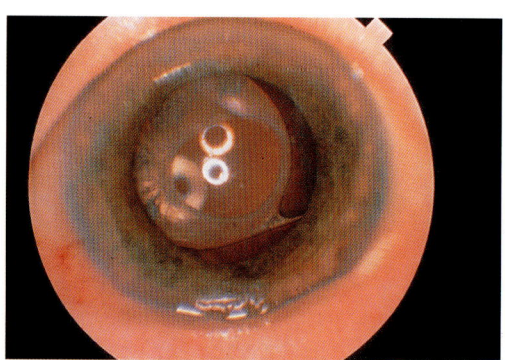

The *most* appropriate management for this patient is

a. continued observation
b. perform multiple radial anterior Nd:YAG capsulotomies
c. perform Nd:YAG posterior capsulotomy
d. increase topical corticosteroid to reduce contraction

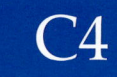 Two years after uncomplicated phacoemulsification with deliberate sulcus placement of a three-piece posterior chamber lens with polypropylene haptics, a healthy adult patient notes intermittent obscurations of vision. Examination during an episode of decreased vision demonstrates a microhyphema and elevation of intraocular pressure to 30 mm Hg. Red reflex examination at the slit lamp reveals the finding shown in the figure.

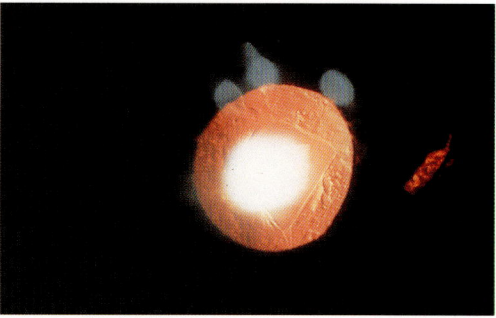

The *most* likely diagnosis is

a. iris neovascularization
b. peripheral uveitis
c. pseudophakic iris chafing syndrome
d. iris nevus syndrome

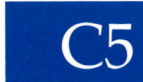

A 23-year-old woman requests refractive surgery. She is a –3.00 myope. Keratometry reading in the right eye is 44.00 D/45.00 D × 90°. Keratometry reading in the left eye is 45.00 D/48.00 D × 120° with +2 distortion of the keratoscopic mires OS.

The *most* appropriate advice to give her is to

a. have radial keratotomy (RK) in the right eye and an RK with transverse incision in the left
b. discontinue her contact lenses indefinitely
c. discontinue her contact lenses for 2 to 3 weeks and return for corneal topography
d. increase artificial tears, since they may help the irregular mires

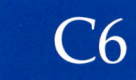

An 18-year-old patient presents with complaints of a decrease in vision for the past several months. Examination shows the eyelids to be thickened, with weeping fissures at the lateral canthi. Slit-lamp examination demonstrates a cataract located anteriorly (see the figure). The patient also complains of multiple skin lesions that are dry, erythematous, and very pruritic.

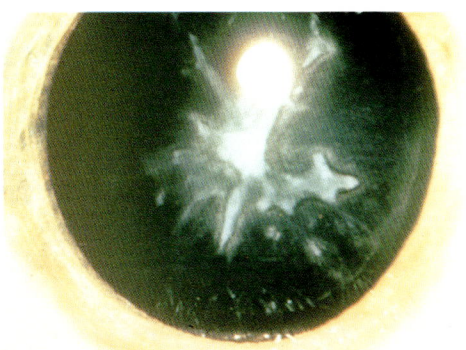

This constellation of findings is *most* characteristic of

a. herpes simplex
b. vernal keratoconjunctivitis
c. atopic disease
d. systemic lupus erythematosus

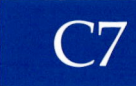

A 65-year-old patient has developed progressive nuclear sclerosis in both eyes and is having difficulty with reading and near work. Refraction is OD –1.25 –1.50 × 155 = 20/50, and OS –5.50 –2.00 × 25 = 20/40. Six years ago he had radial keratotomies performed in both eyes. Prior to his radial keratotomy (RK), he was –5.00 sphere in the right eye and –5.50 sphere in the left eye. He had four-incision RK in each eye with a goal of emmetropia in the right eye and mild myopia in the left eye for near vision. Two years after his RKs, his right eye was 20/60 uncorrected, and his left eye was 20/200. Refraction was OD +2.50 –1.50 × 135 = 20/30; OS –2.75 –0.50 × 180 = 20/30. His original keratometry was OD 42.50 D/43.00 D; OS 42.50 D/43.00 D. His present keratometry is OD 38.50 D/37.50 D; OS 42.00 D/41.50 D. His axial length measurements are OD 25.71 mm and OS 25.94 mm.

The *least* acceptable course of action would be to

a. obtain computerized video keratography of both eyes
b. proceed with the cataract surgery utilizing his present keratometry and axial length measurements
c. calculate his true corneal power by subtracting his refractive effect (original spherical equivalent *minus* two-year post-RK spherical equivalent) from his original keratometry
d. calculate his corneal power by placing a plano contact lens of known curvature on his cornea and refracting over it

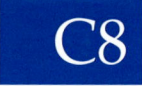

The lens change shown in the figure is often associated with anterior polar cataracts in what associated disease or syndrome?

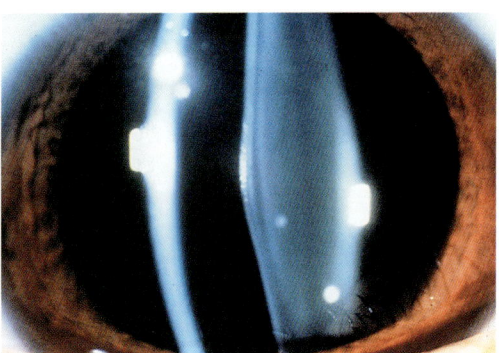

a. Lowe syndrome
b. Alport syndrome
c. rubella
d. Down syndrome

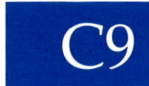 All of the following statements about the rubella syndrome are true *except*

a. The retina often demonstrates a "salt and pepper" appearance.
b. It often includes bilateral nuclear sclerotic cataracts.
c. Virus-induced iridocyclitis may occur if all cortical and nuclear lens material is not removed during the initial cataract surgery.
d. It occurs when the mother is infected during the third trimester.

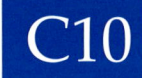 The subtraction video keratograph shown in the figure demonstrates the difference between the preoperative video keratograph (top left, A) and the postoperative video keratograph (bottom left, B). Blue on scale represents little to no dioptric change; red represents significant change.

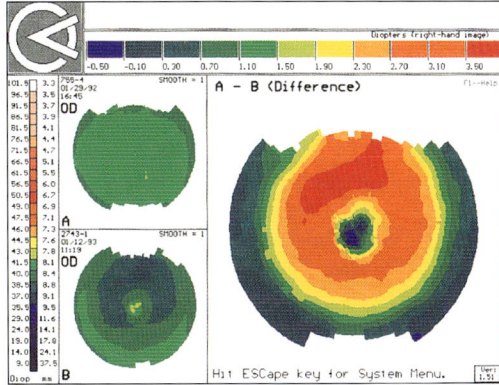

This video keratograph demonstrates

a. central flattening induced by excimer laser photoablation
b. the result of a myopic ablation on a patient with keratoconus
c. a "central island" with a central nipple (steepening) of tissue
d. "bow tie" regular astigmatism

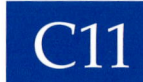

An intraoperative technique is shown in the figure.

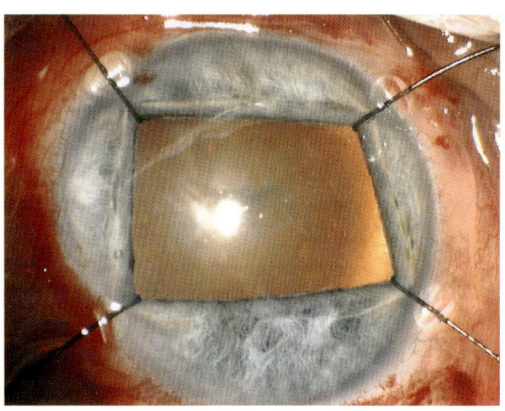

This technique would be *most* advantageous in patients with

a. a dislocated crystalline lens
b. exfoliation syndrome
c. phacolytic glaucoma
d. positive vitreous pressure

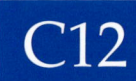

A 32-year-old woman presents with 20/40 vision in both eyes correctable to 20/25 bilaterally and a lens opacity (see the figure).

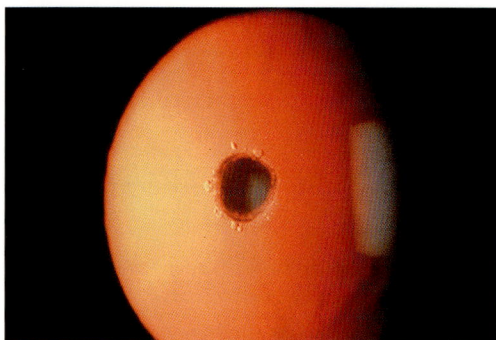

If the lens opacity becomes progressive, which one of the following complications is this patient's eye prone to develop?

a. postoperative uveitis
b. postoperative choroidal detachment
c. intraoperative capsular rupture
d. intraoperative zonular dialysis

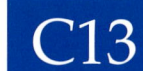

C13 A 25-year-old patient with 6.00 D of preoperative spherical myopia in both eyes is 1 month post eight-incision radial keratotomy (RK) with a 3.0 mm optical zone in the right eye. Her current refractive error is OD −3.75 −2.00 × 175, OS −6.50 −1.00 × 5. Keratometry is 41.75 D/44.50 D × 90° in the right eye. Slit-lamp examination shows excellent depth for the 3 o'clock incision, and approximately 70% for the 9 o'clock incision. The incision depth is difficult to estimate for the other incisions.

The *most* appropriate step would be to

a. perform surgery on her left eye to relieve the anisometropia
b. add eight additional radial keratotomy incisions between the original eight in the right eye
c. obtain computerized video keratography
d. reduce the original optical zone to 2.5 mm with Russian-type out-to-in incisions

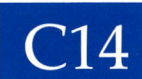

C14 The *most* characteristic type of cataract in retinitis pigmentosa is

a. posterior subcapsular cataract
b. anterior polar cataract
c. nuclear sclerotic cataract
d. cortical spoke cataract

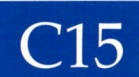

C15 Clear corneal cataract incisions can alter corneal curvature by

a. steepening in the meridian of the incision
b. flattening in the meridian of the incision
c. flattening 90° away from the incision
d. flattening the central cornea

C16 Which statement is *most* correct regarding endothelial cell loss and phacoemulsification?

a. In-situ (within the lens capsule) phacoemulsification takes longer than nuclear tilt posterior chamber and anterior chamber phacoemulsification and, therefore, results in greater endothelial cell loss.
b. Scleral incisions have the same cell loss as corneal incisions.
c. In-situ phacoemulsification causes less cell loss than techniques involving emulsification of the nucleus anterior to the plane of the anterior capsule or iris.
d. Superior and temporal clear-corneal incisions have the same average cell loss.

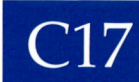

Expected postoperative symptoms in the first week following radial keratotomy include all of the following *except*

a. visual fluctuation
b. starbursting
c. foreign-body sensation
d. metamorphopsia

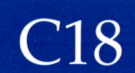

You are asked to examine a 42-year-old engineer who does most of his work at near with a computer. He is a –6.50 D myope. You decide that he is a good candidate for radial keratotomy (RK). He is not worried about having to wear thin glasses but would like to be less dependent on glasses for his near work.

The *most* appropriate optical treatment for his needs would be to

a. fully correct him with RK for emmetropia
b. perform RK and tangential cuts (T-cuts) at 180° to induce with-the-rule cylinder and a multifocal cornea
c. undercorrect him by 1 D in both eyes
d. make him slightly hyperopic in one eye and myopic in the other

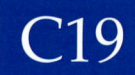

At the conclusion of cataract extraction, an inferior zonular dialysis of approximately 90° is noted. The capsule is otherwise completely intact without a tear or rent. Which of the following statements concerning intraocular lens insertion in this situation is *most* correct?

a. The patient should receive no intraocular lens, since any lens is likely to dislocate.
b. Any appropriate intraocular lens may be inserted into the capsule, and the preferred orientation of the long axis of the implant is horizontal (perpendicular to the axis of the dialysis).
c. A single or multipiece PMMA IOL may be inserted into the ciliary sulcus, and the preferred orientation of the long axis of the implant is vertical (in the axis of the dialysis).
d. A single or multipiece PMMA IOL may be inserted into the ciliary sulcus, and the preferred orientation of the long axis of the implant is horizontal (perpendicular to the axis of the dialysis).

C20 Two years after uncomplicated phacoemulsification performed through a scleral corneal tunnel, the patient is noted to have the complication shown in the figure.

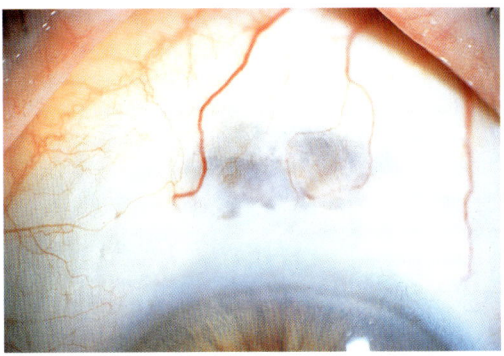

The *most* appropriate course of action at this time would be

a. freehand graft with banked scleral tissue
b. diagnostic workup for a collagen vascular disease
c. suturing of the defect with 10-0 nylon sutures
d. placement of a hydrophilic bandage contact lens

C21 Sunrise syndrome is shown in the figure.

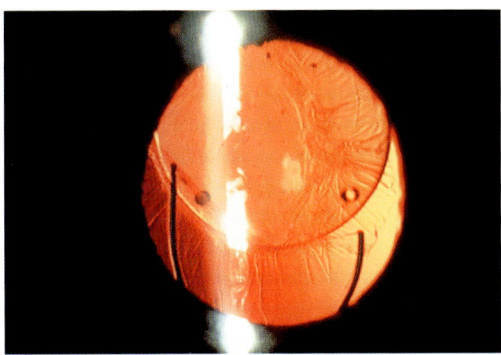

This syndrome is *most* likely caused by

a. an ovoid posterior capsulotomy
b. phacoemulsification of the lens nucleus
c. one lens haptic in the capsular bag and one lens haptic in the ciliary sulcus
d. reduced optic dimension

C22 All of the following statements are true *except*

a. The cornea flattens directly over any sutured incision.
b. The central cornea steepens adjacent to tight limbal sutures.
c. The normal cornea steepens over any incision.
d. Tissue removal produces corneal flattening over the site of tissue removal, whether traumatic or surgically induced.

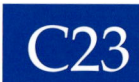 Which of the following statements regarding radial keratotomy (RK) and photorefractive keratectomy (PRK) and regression of effect is *most* accurate?

a. Regression of effect following refractive surgery for myopia implies that the refractive result shifts toward hyperopia. This finding is more profound after PRK.
b. Regression of effect following refractive surgery for myopia implies that the refractive result shifts toward hyperopia. This finding is more profound after RK.
c. Regression of effect following refractive surgery for myopia implies that the refractive result shifts toward myopia. This finding is more profound after PRK.
d. Regression of effect following refractive surgery for myopia implies that the refractive result shifts toward myopia. This finding is more profound after RK.

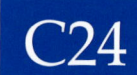 All of the following statements about the advantages of a continuous curvilinear capsulorhexis (CCC) are true *except*

a. It decreases posterior capsular opacification.
b. It makes removal of residual cortex by aspiration easier.
c. It eases and assures in-the-bag IOL implantation.
d. It allows hydrodissection of the nucleus without fear of anterior rim tear extension to the equator.

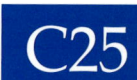 Which of the following statements regarding front-cutting and back-cutting diamond micrometer knives set at *identical* blade depths is true?

a. The front-cutting knife (passed from the limbus toward the center optical zone, or uphill) will achieve a greater depth of cut centrally than the back-cutting knife (passed from the center optical zone to the limbus, or downhill).
b. The back-cutting knife (passed from the center optical zone to the limbus, or downhill) will achieve a greater depth of cut centrally than the front-cutting knife (passed from the limbus toward the center optical zone, or uphill).
c. The knives will achieve equal-depth cuts.
d. Accidental invasion into the center optical zone is more frequent with a back-cutting knife (passed from the optical zone to the limbus) than a front-cutting knife (passed from the limbus toward the optical zone).

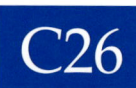 A 50-year-old man with 20/400 uncorrected visual acuity (VA) underwent refractive surgery for a $-4.50 +0.75 \times 96$ refractive error. The surgical plan included a four-incision radial keratotomy with incisions performed at 12, 6, 9, and 3 o'clock and an optical zone of 3.75 mm. At 6 weeks postoperatively, his uncorrected VA was 20/60 with a refraction of $-2.00 +0.75 \times 85$. His manifest VA was 20/15. He desired an enhancement to improve his uncorrected visual acuity. His postoperative corneal topography is shown in the figure.

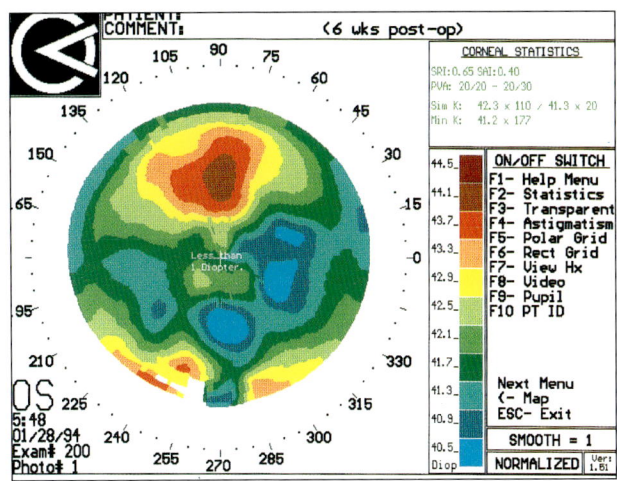

What is the enhancement procedure of choice?

a. The patient is undercorrected (spherical equivalent −1.75 OD) and needs all radial incisions lengthened to decrease the RK optical zone to 3.00 mm.
b. The astigmatism has not been corrected, and tangential cuts (T-cuts) need to be added.
c. The radial incision at 12 o'clock is less effective and needs to be redeepened.
d. The patient is undercorrected with persistent astigmatism and needs radial incisions redeepened and/or lengthened as well as a T-cut at 12 o'clock.

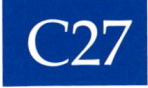

A 37-year-old contact-lens–intolerant patient who is actively involved in scuba diving and skiing and "hates wearing glasses" is interested in refractive surgery. The refractive error in his right eye is −1.25 +2.50 × 75. The refraction in his other eye is similar. He is highly motivated to have his astigmatism corrected.

Which of the following is the most appropriate approach to this patient's needs?

a. Refer him to an excimer laser center.
b. Perform a four-incision radial keratotomy with a 4.0 mm optical zone and two transverse incisions along the 75° axis.
c. Determine the spherical equivalent before planning his surgery.
d. Perform two arcuate incisions in the 165° axis.

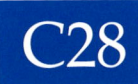

All of the following factors have been shown to affect the outcome of radial keratotomy significantly *except*

a. patient age
b. number of incisions
c. keratometry
d. optical zone diameter

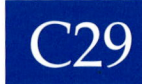 Phacoemulsification is performed after the creation of a continuous, circular capsulotomy. At the completion of nucleus and cortex removal, a radial anterior capsular tear is noted at 6 o'clock, and the posterior capsule appears to be intact.

In this situation, which of the following statements is *least* correct?

a. A multipiece foldable IOL can be placed in the capsular bag.
b. A single-piece (plate) foldable IOL can be placed in the capsular bag.
c. A three-piece or one-piece polymethylmethacrylate (PMMA) IOL can be placed in the capsular bag.
d. A three-piece or one-piece PMMA IOL can be placed in the ciliary sulcus.

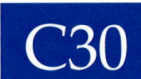 A patient presents with a decrease in vision. As you shake hands with him, you note that his hands have prominent knuckles and short, stubby fingers (see the figure, part A). On ocular examination, you note a mildly cataractous lens shortened in its horizontal and vertical dimensions and slightly increased in its anteroposterior dimension (see the figure, part B). Additionally, the lens is slightly dislocated inferiorly.

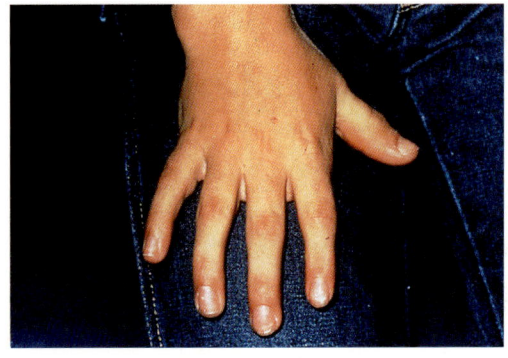
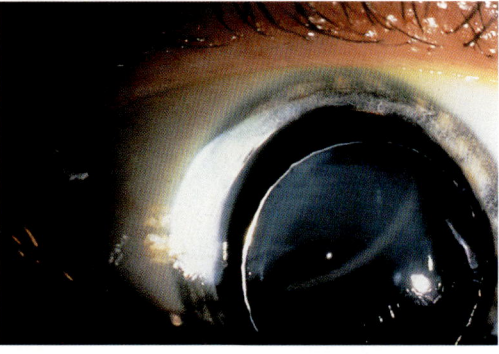
A B

The *most* likely diagnosis is

a. osteogenesis imperfecta
b. Weill-Marchesani syndrome
c. Marfan syndrome
d. homocystinuria

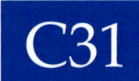 Six weeks after phacoemulsification with implantation of a 12.0 mm overall length single-piece (plate) silicone foldable posterior chamber lens implant, an Nd:YAG laser posterior capsulotomy was performed. Shortly thereafter vision decreased, and the condition shown in the figure was noted on examination.

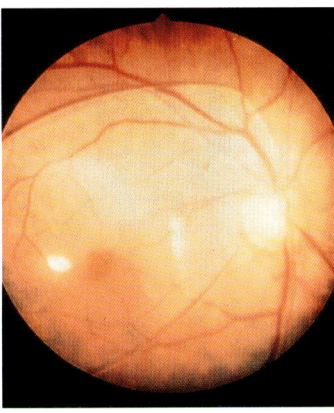

All of the following factors contributed to this finding *except*

a. implant design
b. implant size
c. timing of the capsulotomy
d. intraocular pressure

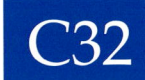 The change shown in the figure was noted during preoperative evaluation for cataract extraction.

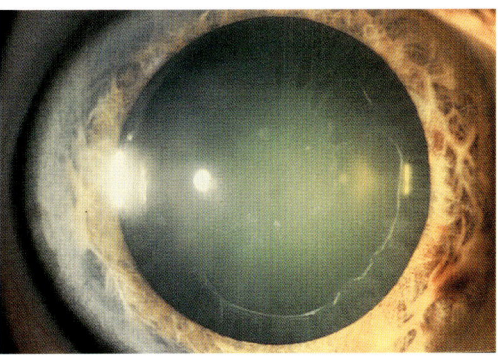

All of the following statements are true *except*

a. The patient is at risk for spontaneous corneal edema following cataract extraction.
b. The patient is at risk for intraoperative zonular dialysis.
c. This condition is associated with an increased incidence of narrow angles.
d. This condition is associated with open-angle glaucoma.

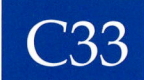 A patient presents with the condition shown in the figure. Following your examination, you decide that the cataract will be removed using a phacoemulsification technique.

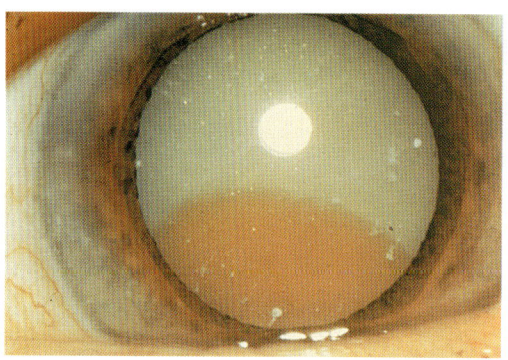

Which of the following steps in the procedure will be the easiest to perform?

a. anterior capsulorhexis
b. nuclear cracking
c. nucleus emulsification
d. aspiration of cortex

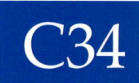 For chemical preparation of the eye prior to ophthalmic surgery, which of the following is *most* effective in decreasing the bacterial flora of the conjunctiva without causing ocular surface toxicity?

a. a mild silver protein solution (Argyrol)
b. 5% (half-strength) povidone-iodine (Betadine) solution
c. 5% (half-strength) povidone-iodine (Betadine) solution followed by irrigation of the conjunctival fornix with saline
d. 5% povidone-iodine (Betadine) scrub/soap

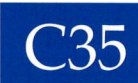 The two posterior chamber intraocular lenses shown in the figure have optics and haptics made of polymethylmethacrylate (PMMA). They are of equal overall length (13.0 mm) and identical power (21.0 D). The only difference between the two lenses is that the optic of the left lens is 5 mm × 6 mm in diameter (oval) and the optic of the right lens is 7.0 mm in diameter (round).

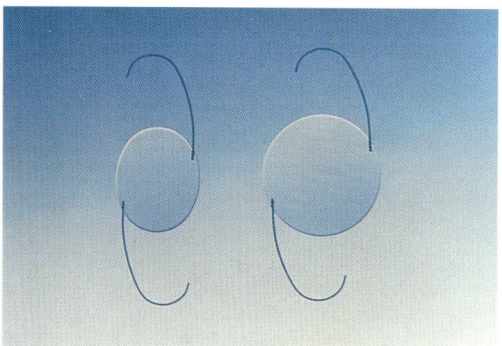

All of the following statements are true *except*

a. The refractive index of these two lens optics is identical.
b. The center thickness of the round lens is greater than that of the oval lens.
c. The center thickness of the oval lens is less than the center thickness of a 6 mm round PMMA optic of the same dioptric power.
d. Both of these lenses will fit into the capsular bag.

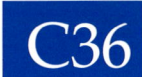

All of the following statements about extracapsular cataract extraction in a patient with diabetes mellitus are true *except*

a. Cataract extraction is highly associated with progression of nonproliferative retinopathy in the operated eye.
b. Patients with preexisting nonproliferative diabetic retinopathy have a worse visual prognosis than those without retinopathy.
c. Overweight women with diabetes have a significantly worse visual outcome than patients with normal body weight and diabetes.
d. The cataract procedure of choice in diabetic patients is a small-incision phacoemulsification in which a 5.0 mm optic IOL is placed through a similarly sized capsulorhexis opening into the capsular bag.

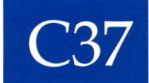

Phacolytic glaucoma is characterized by all of the following *except*

a. a visible break in the lens capsule with inflammation around the lens material
b. a unilateral red eye with diffuse corneal edema
c. an elevated intraocular pressure in the presence of a mature or hypermature cataract
d. a deep anterior chamber with circulating large, white, clumped cells

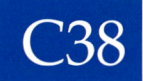

All of the following statements regarding peribulbar anesthesia are true *except*

a. Globe perforation with peribulbar anesthesia is not possible.
b. Peribulbar anesthesia can be performed with needles that are shorter than those that are required for retrobulbar anesthesia.
c. Supplemental anesthesia may be required.
d. Subdural injection is less common with a peribulbar technique than with a retrobulbar technique.

C39 Indications for small-incision phacoemulsification surgery through a temporal clear-corneal incision under topical anesthesia include all of the following *except*

a. a patient on warfarin (Coumadin) therapy for valvular heart disease
b. an uncooperative patient with a history of psychosis
c. a monocular patient with glaucoma and a functioning superior filtering bleb
d. a patient with recurrent but now quiescent cicatricial ocular pemphigoid

C40 All of the following are risk factors in developing an expulsive suprachoroidal hemorrhage *except*

a. axial length greater than or equal to 26.0 mm
b. a history of glaucoma
c. intraoperative pulse greater than or equal to 85 beats per minute
d. an isolated traumatic cataract after remote trauma

C41 Which of the following is *least* likely to be a complication of the procedure shown in the figure?

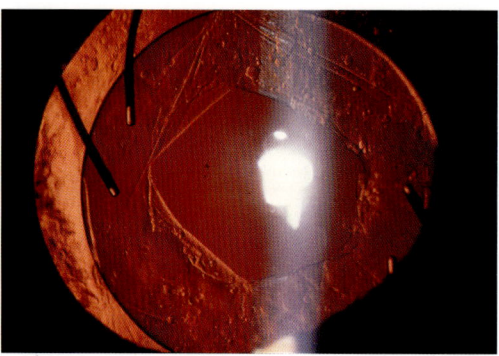

a. increased intraocular pressure
b. acute angle-closure glaucoma
c. retinal detachment
d. cystoid macular edema

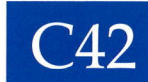

Which of the following statements regarding preoperative testing in a patient with biomicroscopic evidence of cataract is *most* accurate?

a. Contrast sensitivity will help differentiate between visual loss due to the cataract and visual loss from a macular problem.
b. In a patient with good Snellen acuity and complaints of glare, glare testing should be performed as part of the preoperative evaluation.
c. In eyes with opaque media and vision of 20/200 or worse, potential visual acuity testing with interferometry provides an accurate estimate of visual outcome and should be performed.
d. Patients at risk for corneal decompensation from surgery are often difficult to identify through history and clinical examination. Specular microscopy should be routinely performed in patients anticipating cataract extraction by phacoemulsification.

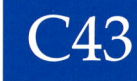

Three months following transscleral fixation of a secondary posterior chamber intraocular lens, the patient returns to your office complaining of foreign-body sensation in the operative eye. Slit-lamp examination reveals the condition shown in the figure below.

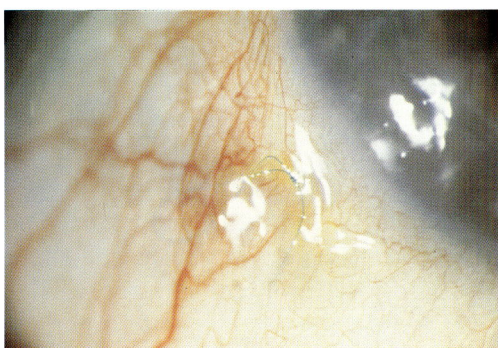

All of the following statements are true *except*

a. This complication could have been avoided if the polypropylene knot and loop had been buried under a scleral flap.
b. This patient is at risk for endophthalmitis.
c. The suture should not be cut and removed, since IOL dislocation would be likely.
d. A return to the operating room is often necessary to rebury the exposed knot or barb.

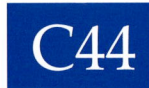
In the early postoperative period, superior corneal edema near the incision and the complication shown in the figure are noted during slit-lamp examination.

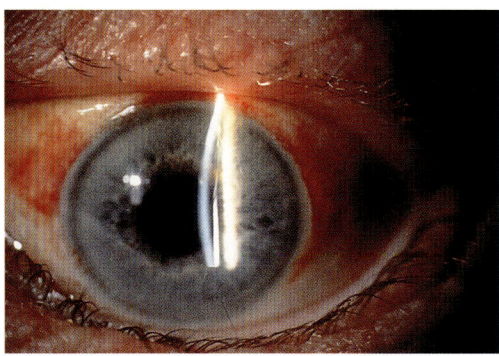

Which of the following is *least* likely to be a cause of this complication?

a. improper introduction of the phacoemulsification tip
b. faulty or difficult insertion of the intraocular lens
c. poor wound closure
d. improper introduction of the irrigation/aspiration tip

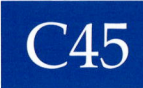
Which of the following statements about refractive surgery is true?

a. Excimer photorefractive keratectomy is effective only for the reduction of myopia.
b. The effect of radial keratotomy decreases with increasing patient age.
c. Keratomileusis in situ (automated lamellar keratectomy, or ALK) can effectively reduce myopia and hyperopia.
d. Astigmatic arcuate incisions cause an overall flattening of the cornea and hence reduce not only astigmatism but also myopia.

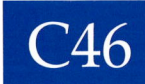
During phacoemulsification a capsular break is noted with vitreous in the anterior chamber. Nucleus removal is incomplete. All of the following steps should be taken *except*

a. continue gentle phacoemulsification, since the phacoemulsification instrument efficiently cuts vitreous
b. inject viscoelastic beneath the nuclear remnant to keep it elevated
c. consider conversion to an extracapsular procedure with utilization of a lens loop to remove the nuclear fragment
d. remove all vitreous from the anterior chamber using an automated vitrector and low inflow

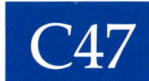

C47 All of the following are signs of a posterior capsular rupture during phacoemulsification *except*

a. constriction of the pupil
b. slight deepening of the anterior chamber
c. the appearance of vitreous in the anterior chamber
d. an area of the posterior capsule that appears "too clear" compared to adjacent areas

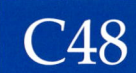

C48 A scleral-pocket incision and closure (which enters the anterior chamber anterior to Schwalbe's line) is shown in the figure.

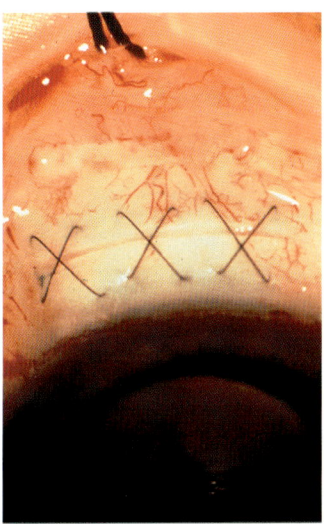

This technique would be expected to produce

a. transient keratometric steepening in the surgical meridian
b. transient keratometric flattening in the surgical meridian
c. transient keratometric steepening 90° away from the surgical meridian
d. emmetropia

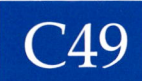

C49 All of the following are components of one or more of the commercially available viscoelastic materials *except*

a. sodium hyaluronate
b. chondroitin sulfate
c. hydroxypropylmethylcellulose
d. keratan sulfate

When comparing radial keratotomy (RK) to excimer laser photorefractive keratectomy (PRK), which of the following statements is *most* accurate?

a. PRK is more predictable than RK in the −1 D to −4 D myopic range.
b. PRK flattens the central cornea and RK steepens the central cornea.
c. Reading glasses are needed less often in presbyopic patients undergoing PRK as compared to RK.
d. Early postoperative vision is worse and pain more significant following PRK as compared to RK.

SECTION FOUR
Neuro-Ophthalmology

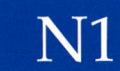

A 65-year-old woman presents with acute visual loss OD and periocular ache. The results of her examination are as follows:

Best-corrected acuity: 20/40 OD, 20/20 OS
Ishihara color plates: 9/10 correct OD, 10/10 correct OS
Pupils: 5 mm OU and round, + RAPD OD
Motility: Normal, no proptosis
Visual fields: OD shown in the figure; OS normal
Fundi: Optic disc swollen OD, normal OS

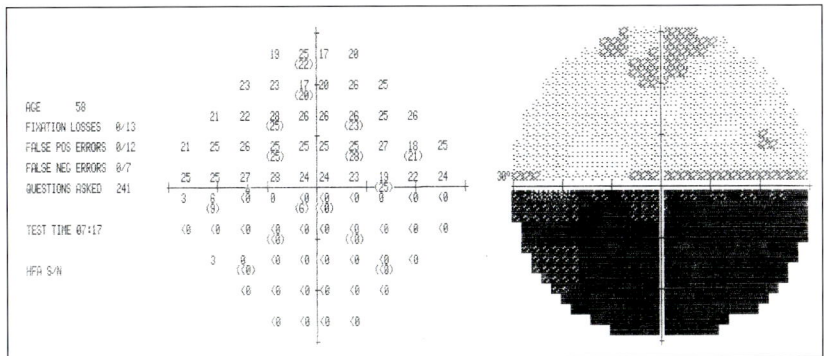

What is the *most* appropriate diagnostic test to perform *immediately*?

a. CT scan of the orbits (axial and coronal, with 1 mm to 2 mm sections, with contrast)
b. fluorescein angiography
c. MRI of the head with gadolinium and of the orbits with fat suppression
d. erythrocyte sedimentation rate

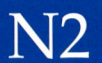

In a patient who has acute optic neuritis in the right eye, which of the following is true?

a. There must be a relative afferent pupillary defect present in the right eye.
b. There cannot be a better pupillary response in the right eye than in the left.
c. It would be rare for the patient to have a new visual field defect on automated perimetry in the left eye.
d. With the information given, the results of the relative afferent pupillary defect test cannot be predicted.

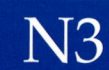

N3 An emergent consultation is requested on a comatose man with significant periocular trauma to the right eye. A CT scan of the head is essentially normal. The patient's pupils are 8 mm OD, 4 mm OS; the right pupil does not react to direct light. The right eye is exodeviated and has complete ptosis, and oculocephalic maneuver indicates that the right eye does not cross the midline in the field of action of the right medial rectus muscle. There is no enophthalmos or proptosis. Intraocular pressures are 19 mm Hg OD and 12 mm Hg OS. Both fundi are unremarkable.

For the purpose of guiding emergent treatment, which of the following is the *most* appropriate test to perform?

a. a CT scan of the orbits
b. forced duction of the right eye
c. examination of the relative magnitude of the pupillary response of the left eye when the left and then the right eye is illuminated
d. a pattern visual evoked response

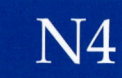

N4 A 20-year-old woman presents with pupils of unequal size. The examination is normal but for the pupillary examination, which reveals:

Dim light: 8 mm OD, 4 mm OS
Bright light: 8 mm OD, 2 mm OS
Near fixation: 8 mm OD, 1.5 mm OS

What is the *most* appropriate sequence of pharmacologic testing to perform on the patient?

a. 1% pilocarpine, 2.5% methacholine (Mecholyl)
b. 0.05% pilocarpine, 1% pilocarpine
c. 5% cocaine, 1% hydroxyamphetamine (Paredrine)
d. 1% hydroxyamphetamine (Paredrine), 0.5% phenylephrine

N5 A 22-year-old woman exhibits a dilated right pupil that you clinically suspect is an Adie's tonic pupil. The pupils are 8 mm OD, 5 mm OS in dim light, and 8 mm OD, 2 mm OS in bright light. The motility is normal, and there is no ptosis. While preparing the appropriate pharmacologic solutions, you take a more detailed history.

Which of the following historical points would be of the *least* significance in a patient who demonstrates a large pupil that does not constrict?

a. The patient is an ICU nurse who runs cardiac resuscitation codes.
b. The patient is aware of an inability to read with the right eye only.
c. The patient says that the right eye with the larger pupil has always had a lighter colored iris than the left eye.
d. The patient has a history of motion sickness and has just returned from a cruise.

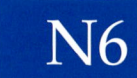 An 8-year-old girl is brought in by her mother because of difficulty reading. The mother mentions that the child has a chronic "cold in the eye" because both eyes are always red (see the figures). The vision is 20/20 OU at near and at distance; the pupils and fundi are normal. You also notice that the child has difficulty moving her eyes in the horizontal plane, and that this paresis is overcome by the oculocephalic maneuver.

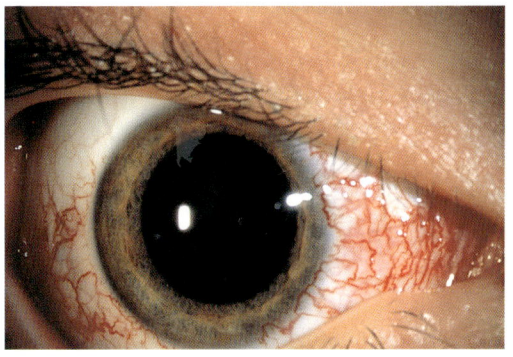
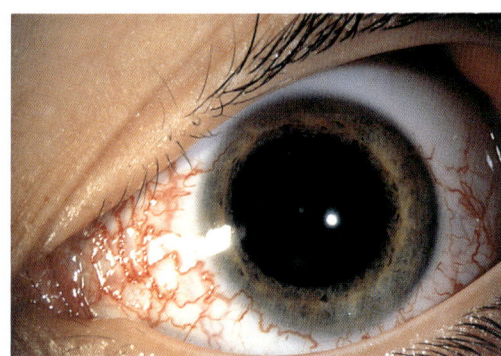

A   B

Based upon the presentation and the external eye appearance, what is the *most* appropriate course of action?

a. Prescribe a trial of topical sulfa-corticosteroid combination for 2 weeks.
b. Inquire if the child has missed her early developmental milestones.
c. Inquire if the child is often sick and is more clumsy lately.
d. Prescribe a course of oral trimethoprim-sulfamethoxazole (Bactrim) for 3 weeks.

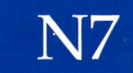 A man presents after having fallen off a scaffold 20 feet from the ground. He had loss of consciousness for an hour and is still lethargic. He has an orbital roof fracture on the right and a temporal bone fracture on the left. Because of lethargy, the patient's acuity cannot adequately be assessed. His pupils are 6 mm OU, round, reactive to light, with a trace relative afferent pupillary defect OD. The motility shows a 2+ underaction of the right lateral rectus, right medial rectus, inferior rectus, and inferior oblique muscles. There is 2 mm ptosis OD. The right eye's external appearance is shown in the figure; the left eye is normal externally. The right fundus shows venous distention but is otherwise normal.

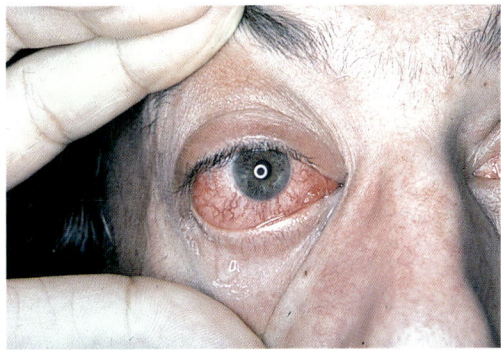

All of the following would be consistent with the clinical presentation *except*

a. 4 mm of proptosis of the right eye
b. intraocular pressures of 14 mm Hg OD and 24 mm Hg OS
c. ocular bruit OD
d. depressed corneal reflex OD

N8 A 65-year-old woman presents with double vision, which has been present for 3 weeks. She has had good general health until she recently developed an arrhythmia. Although her internist placed her on oral procainamide for this arrhythmia 3 months ago, she has continued to feel weak and tired; the internist, who has already obtained a negative MRI of the head with gadolinium, has referred her to you. Her ocular and neurologic examinations are normal except for her horizontal eye movements, which are shown in the figures. She thinks that her right eye becomes "more droopy" in the evening.

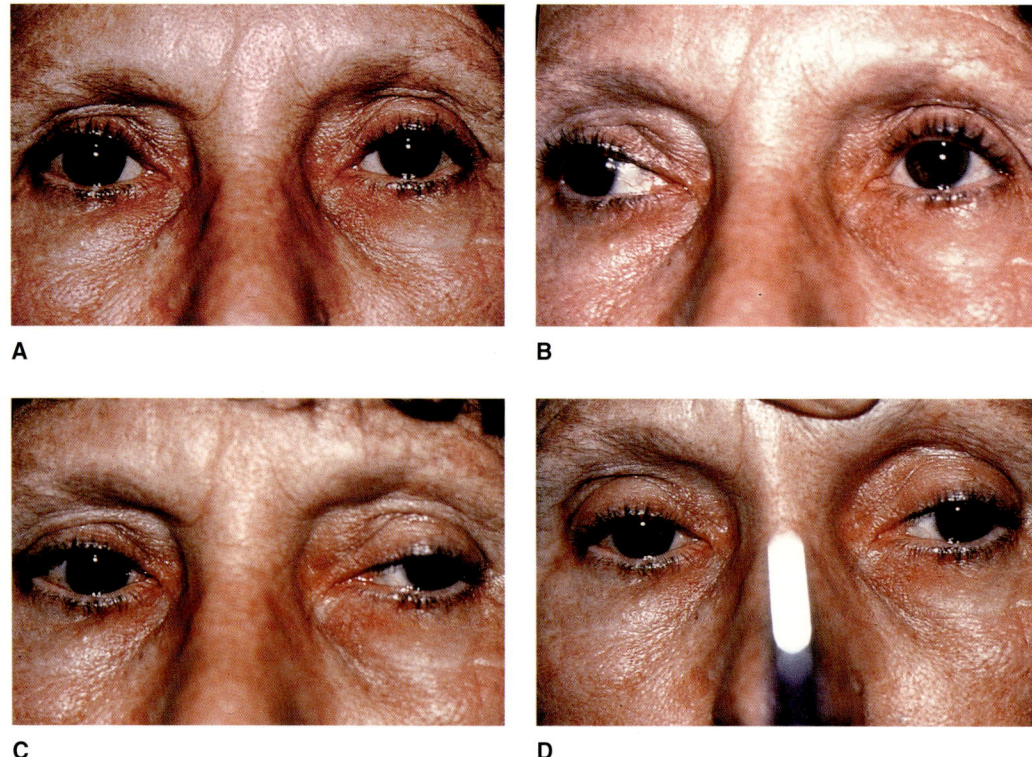

Which of the following points is *most* relevant in arriving at the patient's ultimate diagnosis and a treatment plan?

a. She has taken 50,000 units of vitamin A daily for 6 weeks.
b. Discuss with the internist whether another agent is available for her arrhythmia therapy.
c. The diplopia is more noticeable when she reads than when she performs distance tasks.
d. She is allergic to penicillin.

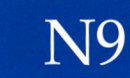

A patient is brought to the emergency room comatose with a head injury from a motor vehicle accident. He has no other medical problems. In your initial evaluation, the pupillary responses are normal, and there is no relative afferent pupillary defect (RAPD). One hour later, after the neurosurgery service finishes its evaluation and you reevaluate the patient, the pupils are 4 mm OU, and a 4+ RAPD is seen in the left eye. The intraocular pressure is 16 mm Hg OD, and 42 mm Hg OS. The external examination reveals mild chemosis and 4 mm of proptosis OS. The neurosurgeon asks you not to dilate the pupils because the patient is comatose and she wishes to observe the pupils for dilation indicative of cerebral herniation. The right fundus is normal; the left cannot be visualized. The orbital CT scan is shown in the figure.

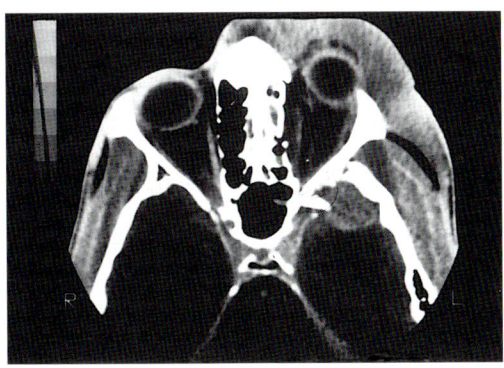

All of the following are a part of an appropriate treatment plan *except*

a. performing a right lateral canthotomy
b. administering intravenous megadose corticosteroids (at least 1 g of methylprednisolone or equivalent daily)
c. planning with the orbital surgeon and neurosurgeon for possible optic canal and optic nerve sheath exploration and/or decompression if the neuro-ophthalmic examination shows no improvement and the patient is cleared for the operating room
d. starting no therapy and reevaluating the patient in 48 hours with a dilated fundus examination

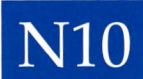

Based on the data generated by the Optic Neuritis Treatment Trial, which of the following is true about the management of patients with acute unilateral optic neuritis?

a. Patients should be treated with intravenous corticosteroids because they demonstrated significantly better visual acuity performance at 1 year than did patients treated with placebo therapy.
b. All patients with an acute optic neuritis should be treated with intravenous corticosteroids.
c. MRI should be performed on a patient with acute unilateral optic neuritis with no history of prior neurologic disease.
d. Patients with acute unilateral optic neuritis should be treated with oral prednisone to diminish the frequency of subsequent attacks of optic neuritis.

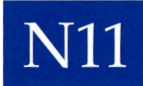

N11

A 22-year-old woman presents with acute optic neuritis OS of 1 day's duration. Her past medical history and neurologic examination are normal. The results of her ophthalmic examination are as follows:

Best-corrected acuity: 20/20 OD, 20/40 OS

Ishihara color plates: 10/10 correct OD, 3/10 correct OS

Pupils: 7 mm OU, round and reactive; 3+ RAPD OS

Motility: Normal

Slit lamp: Normal

Intraocular pressures: Normal

Visual fields: Normal OD, 10° central scotoma OS

Fundi: Normal OD, trace hyperemic swelling OS, no hemorrhages or exudates

Which of the following is the *most* appropriate sequence of management steps in this patient?

a. Obtain a chest x-ray, treat with 250 mg q6h methylprednisolone sodium succinate (Solumedrol) IV for 3 days, followed by 11 days of oral prednisone.
b. Obtain antinuclear antibody (ANA) and a chest x-ray; if ANA is positive, treat with oral prednisone, 80 mg/day for 2 weeks.
c. Obtain MRI the next morning, and see the patient in the afternoon after the scan is completed.
d. Begin the patient on 80 mg/day of prednisone while awaiting results of MRI.

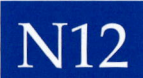

N12

A patient presents with gradual visual loss in both eyes over 3 weeks. The results of the examination are as follows:

Best-corrected acuity: 20/20 OU

Pupils: 5 mm OU, round and reactive; 1+ RAPD OD

Motility: Normal

Slit lamp: Normal

Intraocular pressures: 12 mm Hg OD, 14 mm Hg OS

Visual fields: Shown in the figures

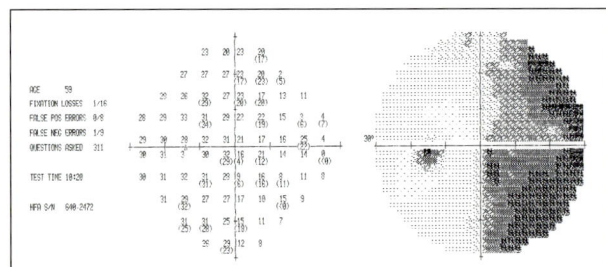

A

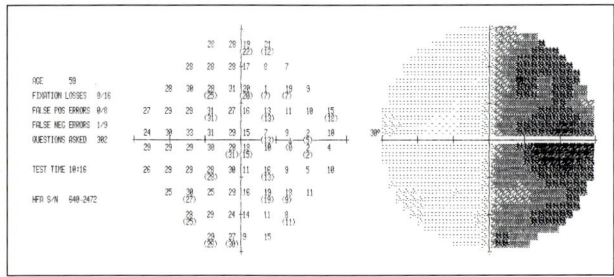

B

Which of the following statements is true?

a. Two lesions are required to cause this presentation.
b. A lesion in the left anterior-most occipital lobe could cause this presentation.
c. If followed over time, this patient will not develop any optic atrophy.
d. The lesion is in the left optic tract.

N13 A 10-year-old boy is examined for bilateral progressive visual loss that has occurred over 1 month. He has polyuria and polydipsia and is found to have diabetes insipidus.

Which of the following is the *most* likely associated visual field deficit?

a. a unilateral nasal step
b. a bilateral nasal defect respecting the midline
c. a complete left homonymous hemianopsia
d. a bilateral temporal defect respecting the midline, denser in the inferior quadrants

N14 The figures show the MRI results of a child with the same histologic lesion as the child in Question N13 but in another location.

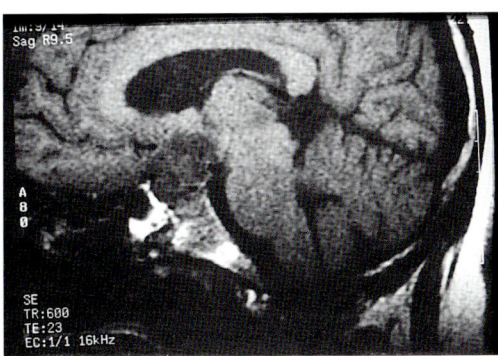
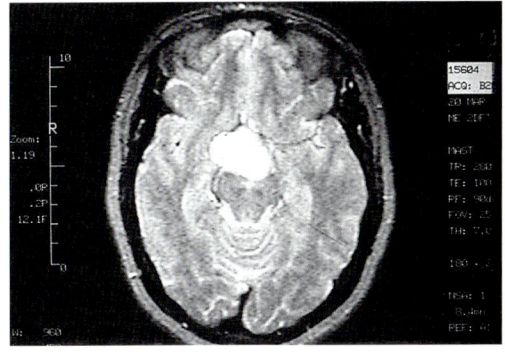

A   B

(A) T1-weighted MRI, sagittal projection, without gadolinium. **(B)** T2-weighted MRI, axial projection.

What is the *most* likely pathology of the lesion shown?

a. pituitary adenoma
b. meningioma
c. craniopharyngioma
d. anterior communicating artery aneurysm

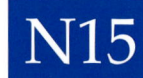

A 17-year-old boy receives an ophthalmic examination before beginning driver's education. The results of the examination are as follows:

Uncorrected acuity: 20/20 OU

Pupils: 5 mm OU, round and reactive; mild RAPD OD

Motility: Normal

Slit lamp: Normal

Intraocular pressures: 16 mm Hg OD, 18 mm Hg OS

Visual fields: Inferior altitudinal defect OD, normal OS

All of the following points in the history or examination, if elicited, would aid in arriving at a diagnosis *except*

a. He has optic nerve hypoplasia OD, and his mother has insulin-dependent (juvenile-onset) diabetes mellitus.
b. A cilioretinal artery is present OD only.
c. The patient had an episode of marked acute visual loss OD with pain on ocular rotation 2 years before, with partial recovery.
d. A superior hemiretinal detachment is present OD.

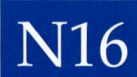

All of the following statements about optokinetic response testing are true *except*

a. Absence of response with the tape moving to the patient's left may indicate a left frontal lobe lesion.
b. Absence of response with the tape moving to the patient's right may indicate a right parietal lesion.
c. Presence of optokinetic nystagmus response to an optokinetic drum at a test distance of 3 feet indicates a visual acuity of 20/60 or better.
d. In a patient with a complete right adduction deficit, ability to cause the right eye to fully adduct in response to an optokinetic drum indicates that the ophthalmoparesis is not infranuclear in origin.

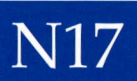

A patient involved in a motor vehicle accident had loss of consciousness for 10 minutes. She has an abduction deficit of the right eye, with only about 10% of normal amplitude of abduction beyond the midline remaining. The anterior examination is normal; exophthalmometry readings are symmetric.

Which of the following would be consistent with the presence of a right sixth-nerve palsy *without* an entrapped medial rectus?

a. restriction of the right eye on forced abduction, no force generated with attempted abduction on forced generation test
b. ability to induce full abduction OD with oculocephalic maneuver
c. no restriction on forced abduction OD, diminished force generated with attempted abduction on forced generation test
d. exodeviation on right gaze

N18 A 68-year-old man complains only of recent onset of "trouble reading." There is no past medical history. The results of the patient's examination are as follows:

Best-corrected acuity: Distance—20/25 OU; near—20/20 OU

Pupils: 3 mm OU, round and reactive; no RAPD

Lid fissures: 10 mm OU

Motility: Horizontal eye movements normal, volitional down gaze severely and symmetrically limited, up gaze mildly limited. Oculocephalic maneuver completely overcomes the vertical eye movement deficiency.

Slit lamp: Normal

Intraocular pressures: Normal

Visual fields: Normal

Fundi: Normal

The *most* likely diagnosis is

a. botulism
b. myasthenia gravis
c. congenital fibrosis syndrome
d. progressive supranuclear palsy (Steele-Richardson-Olszewski syndrome)

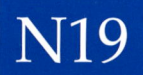

N19 Which of the following would be *most* inconsistent with the diagnosis of the patient in Question N18?

a. extensor neck rigidity
b. dementia
c. pigmentary retinopathy
d. square wave jerks

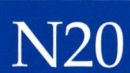

N20 A 3-year-old girl is brought in by her mother for evaluation of a mass that is medial and superior to the left medial canthus and that has been present since birth. The mother is not sure if it has been growing. The examination is normal except for nystagmus OU. You have difficulty visualizing the fundus. The child is short for her age; otherwise, she is doing well.

Appropriate management at this point includes all of the following *except*

a. examination under anesthesia
b. neuroimaging
c. pediatric endocrinologic consultation
d. needle biopsy of the mass, followed by neuroimaging if not inflammatory

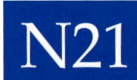 Which of the following conditions is the *most* likely explanation for the visual fields shown in the figures?

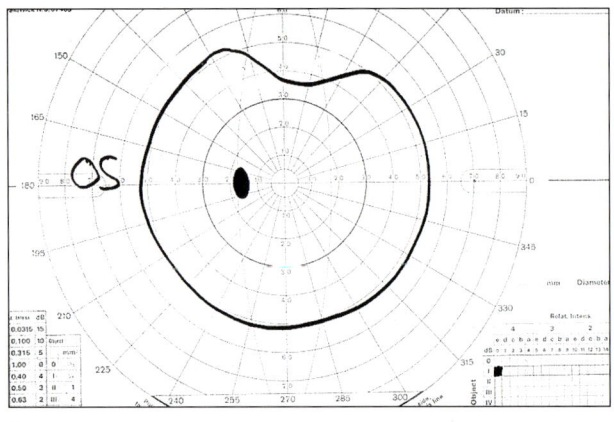
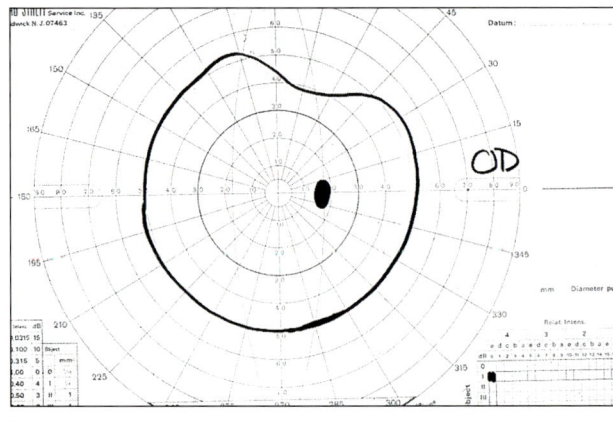

A   B

a. pituitary adenoma
b. tilted optic nerve heads
c. bilateral optic nerve pits
d. craniopharyngioma

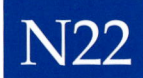 A 335-pound 25-year-old woman comes in on a Monday for evaluation of bilateral synchronous visual obscurations lasting 15 seconds. These have been occurring for 3 weeks. She has no other medical history and is on no medications. Her examination is normal except for enlarged blind spots on visual field testing and marked bilateral papilledema.

What is the *most* reasonable next step in her management?

a. Obtain an MRI that day; if it is negative, begin her on acetazolamide 500 mg q6h and see her in 3 days to determine whether the papilledema has improved.
b. Obtain an MRI on her that day; if it is negative, arrange for a spinal tap shortly thereafter.
c. Start her on acetazolamide 500 mg q6h, and refer her to a neurologist on Thursday.
d. Put her on a weight-reduction and salt-restriction diet, start her on acetazolamide 500 mg q6h, and see her in 4 days to determine whether the papilledema has improved and to reassess the visual function.

N23 Which of the following is true about Leber's hereditary optic neuropathy?

a. It is purely a clinical diagnosis, based on the family inheritance pattern.
b. Females may develop Leber's hereditary optic neuropathy.
c. It is rare for affected patients to have no family history of visual loss.
d. The onset in the two eyes is always simultaneous.

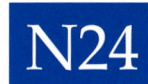

A 70-year-old man presents with a 7-day history of diplopia, having just been discharged from the hospital by his neurologist. He is referred to you to see if prism glasses are indicated. He has a complete right pupil-involving third-nerve palsy. The neurologist tells you that his examination is otherwise normal. The patient says that since he has had the double vision, he has also had a headache with loss of appetite. The results of the evaluation performed by the neurologist are as follows:

MRI with gadolinium: Normal

Lumbar puncture: Normal

Cerebral angiography: Normal

Edrophonium (Tensilon) test: Normal

Acetylcholine receptor antibody: Normal

Glucose tolerance test: Normal

Syphilis and Lyme serologies: Normal

Blood count, ANA, rheumatoid factor: Normal

The results of your examination of the patient are as follows:

Best-corrected acuity: 20/40 OD, 20/30 OS

Ishihara color plates: Normal OU

Pupils: Dim—8 mm OD, 7 mm OS; light—8 mm OD, 2 mm OS; near—8 mm OD, 2 mm OS

Lid fissures: 0 mm OD, 10 mm OS

Motility: 4+ underaction of right inferior oblique, inferior rectus, superior rectus, and medial rectus muscles; lateral rectus muscle intact, incyclotorsion present. Motility of left eye normal. No aberrant regeneration is seen.

Prism cover test: At distance, exotropia = 25 prism diopters; at near, exotropia = 35 prism diopters

Slit lamp: Normal

Intraocular pressures: Normal

Media: 2+ nuclear sclerotic cataract OD, 1+ nuclear sclerotic cataract OS

Fundi: Normal

Which of the following is the *most* important and appropriate immediate step in the management of this patient?

a. Repeat the edrophonium (Tensilon) test with a prism cover test.
b. Obtain an erythrocyte sedimentation rate.
c. Give him 10 base-in ground-in prism in front of the OD for distance, and give him a 25 prism diopter Fresnel prism base-in for near.
d. Give him a patch to use as needed.

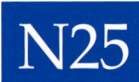

A 9-year-old girl is brought in by her father, a pediatrician. She has had six episodes that are extremely similar, one every 4 weeks; he took pictures of the last episode (see the figures). She becomes cranky and lethargic, and 1 day later, gets the ophthalmoparesis shown in the figures. Her pupils are 6 mm OU in dim light, 3 mm in bright light, round and reactive to light, with no RAPD. There are no other neurologic signs. As soon as the ophthalmoparesis begins, she feels better. The ophthalmoparesis lasts 1 week. Once it resolves, her examination results return to normal. The father has already obtained MRI and a high-resolution magnetic resonance angiogram, which are both normal.

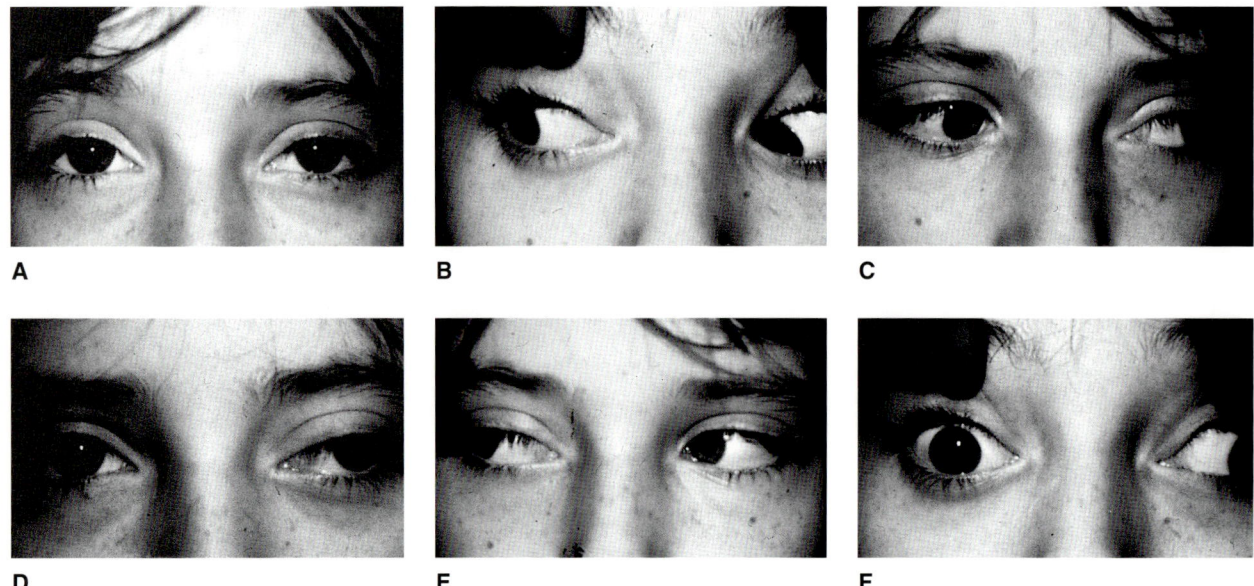

Eye movements of a 9-year-old girl. Before episode: **(A)** Primary gaze; **(B)** right gaze; **(C)** left gaze. During episode: **(D)** Primary gaze; **(E)** right gaze; **(F)** left gaze.

Which of the following is the *most* appropriate management step?

a. Perform a neostigmine (Prostigmin) test.
b. Obtain a spinal tap.
c. Start her on pyridostigmine bromide (Mestinon), 30 mg q4–6h.
d. Begin a trial of propranolol (Inderal) or amitriptyline (Elavil) determined as appropriate for her age and size by her pediatrician father.

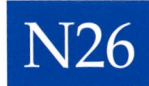

N26 A 45-year-old right-handed male executive who is an avid golfer presents with the complaint that for the past year, whenever he addresses a golf ball, it appears to be shimmering up and down, with perhaps a rotatory component to it. Sometimes the ball looks double to him in the vertical plane. The patient, a good observer, says that the image moves and is double only when viewed with the right eye. The results of his examination are normal.

Which of the following is the *most* appropriate action to take?

a. Start the patient on carbamazepine (Tegretol).
b. Obtain a psychiatric consultation.
c. Start the patient on phenytoin (Dilantin).
d. Perform an edrophonium (Tensilon) test.

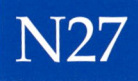

N27 A 67-year-old Asian man consulted you 3 months ago with an isolated right sixth-nerve palsy that had been present for 3 months. His CT scan with contrast of the head, edrophonium (Tensilon) test, glucose tolerance test, sedimentation rate, and serologies for Lyme disease and syphilis were normal. He now presents with a left sixth-nerve palsy to accompany the persistent right sixth-nerve palsy. The results of the rest of the examination remain normal. There is no proptosis. A spinal tap performed by his neurologist 1 day earlier was normal.

The *most* likely location of the pathologic process is

a. bilateral abducens nucleus
b. both orbital apices
c. genu of right facial nerve around abducens nucleus
d. clivus

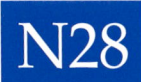

N28 In the patient in Question N27, which of the following is the *least* important in terms of his management plan?

a. Obtain MRI of the base of the brain.
b. Obtain an otolaryngology consult.
c. Perform another spinal tap in a few days.
d. Obtain cervical carotid ultrasonography.

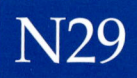 A 56-year-old woman presents with a history of 12 months of double vision and 6 months of ptosis OS. She says that her vision is normal in each eye, and that she has no pain. Her past medical history is normal. The results of her examination are as follows:

Best-corrected acuity: 20/20 OU

Ishihara color plates: Normal OU

Pupils: 5 mm OU, round and reactive; no RAPD

Lid fissures: 10 mm OD, 7 mm OS

Corneal reflex: Depressed OS; rest of trigeminal function remarkable for decreased cutaneous sensation in the distribution of the left maxillary nerve.

Motility: Normal OD; OS 3+ underaction of lateral rectus muscle; 1+ underaction of left medial, superior, and inferior rectus muscles; trace underaction of left inferior oblique muscle; superior oblique muscle normal.

Exophthalmometry: Base 103 mm, OD 18 mm, OS 20 mm

Slit lamp: Mild superficial punctate staining OS, otherwise normal

Intraocular pressures: 14 mm Hg OU, normal pulse pressure

Visual fields: Normal

Fundi: Normal

The *most* likely location of the lesion is

a. limited to the left cavernous sinus, sparing the chiasm
b. involving the left cavernous sinus and the chiasm
c. limited to the left orbital apex
d. left maxillary sinus

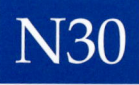 With the presentation and the MRI scans (shown below) from the patient in Question N29, what is the likely underlying pathophysiology?

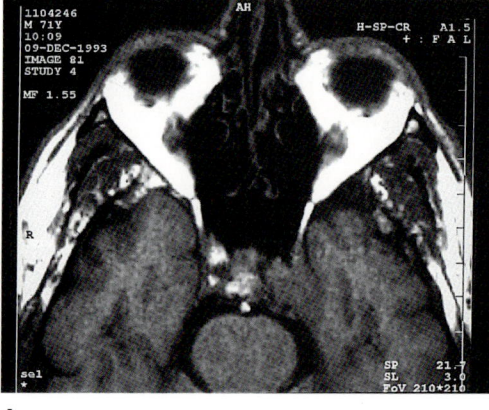
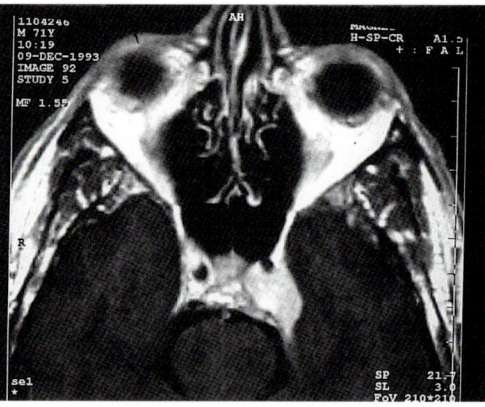

A
B

a. meningioma
b. Tolosa-Hunt syndrome
c. dysthyroid ophthalmopathy
d. pituitary apoplexy

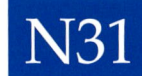

A 57-year-old woman comes for a routine periodic examination to have her reading glasses changed. She has no complaints. Your screening protocol includes a visual field examination that shows a normal field OS and an inferior field defect OD (see the figures). The results of the rest of the examination are as follows:

Best-corrected acuity: 20/20 OU

Ishihara color plates: Normal OU

Pupils: 4 mm OU, round and reactive; 1+ RAPD OD

Motility: Normal

Exophthalmometry: Base 98 mm, OD 19 mm, OS 18 mm

Slit lamp: Normal

Intraocular pressures: Normal

Fundi: Mild disc edema OD, normal OS

The patient denies pain. Because of the findings, you elect to obtain an imaging study. What is the *most* appropriate study to request?

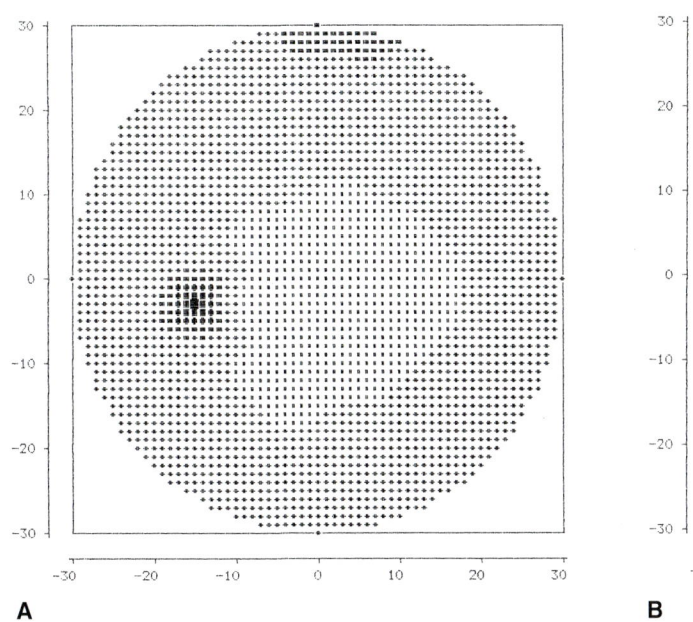
A

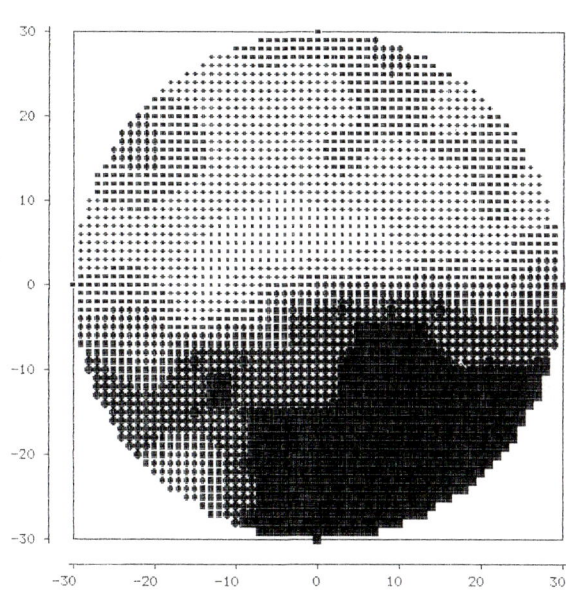
B

a. CT scan of the orbit, without contrast
b. MRI of the brain, with gadolinium
c. CT scan of the head, with contrast
d. MRI of the orbit/optic nerves, with gadolinium and fat-suppression sequences

N32 The figures show the MRI results for the patient in Question N31. Part A is a T1 weighted image without contrast; part B is a T1, fat-suppressed, gadolinium-enhanced image.

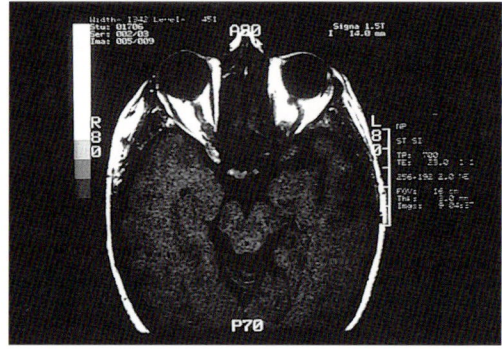
A

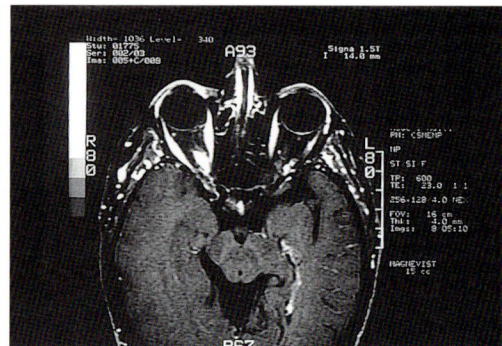
B

Given the presentation and the MRI results, what is now the *most* appropriate management of this patient?

a. Perform a biopsy of the optic nerve.
b. Perform a CT scan of the optic nerve with contrast.
c. Do nothing now and reexamine the patient in 2 months; if still stable, see again in a few months, with a repeat MRI at 6 months.
d. Give a diagnostic and therapeutic course of corticosteroids.

N33 The patient in Question N31 returns for her 6-month followup. At the previous visit, her examination was unchanged from the initial evaluation. Her visual acuity OD has now dropped to 20/60; the color plates are now 4/10 correct OD; the afferent pupillary defect is more apparent; and an optociliary shunt vessel is now seen on the right disc. The visual field defect is also worse, with a central scotoma breaking out into the old inferior scotoma.

What is the *most* appropriate next course of action?

a. Repeat the MRI; if no change, see the patient again in 4 months.
b. Repeat the MRI; if no growth, resect the lesion.
c. Repeat the MRI; irradiate the lesion.
d. Obtain a CT scan of the optic nerves to see if any calcifications have developed.

N34 Which of the following historical points or physical findings would *most* call for MRI in a patient who is having an eleventh bout of a classic migraine syndrome?

a. The patient is 17 years old.
b. The patient is a male.
c. Hemianopia is always on the same side.
d. The visual phenomena are homonymous.

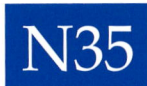

N35 A patient presents with optic neuropathy and uveitis with mutton-fat keratic precipitates. The patient is noted to have bilateral large, nodular lacrimal glands and a white raised lesion on the involved optic nerve head.

Which of the following test results would be *most* likely to exclude the diagnosis of sarcoidosis in this patient?

a. a normal chest x-ray
b. a normal ACE (angiotensin converting enzyme)
c. a normal conjunctival biopsy
d. a positive PPD (purified protein derivative), with the rest of the anergy panel negative (normal cutaneous response was present to mumps)

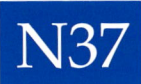

N36 All of the following syndromes with neuro-ophthalmic signs are associated with the endocrinopathy mentioned *except*

a. chiasmal trauma/diabetes insipidus
b. de Morsier's syndrome/growth failure
c. angiomatosis retinae (von Hippel-Lindau disease)/pheochromocytoma
d. chiasmal sarcoidosis/Cushing's disease

N37 A 37-year-old woman presents with ptosis and ophthalmoplegia. She first noted ptosis at age 12, and noted trouble moving her eyes 3 years later. It has been progressive over the years; she never had any diplopia, and she believes that her vision, once her eyelids are raised, is normal. There is no family history. She denies other medical problems, and she has not seen a physician for 10 years. The results of her examination are as follows:

Uncorrected acuity: 20/20 OU

Ishihara color plates: Normal OU

Pupils: 4 mm OU, round and reactive; no RAPD

Lid fissures: 2 mm OU

Orbicularis tone: Mild symmetric weakness

Ocular rotations: Complete ophthalmoplegia, not overcome by oculocephalic (doll's head) maneuver or Bell's phenomenon

Neck: No rigidity

Fundi: Discs sharp and pink, questionable slight "salt and pepper" appearance to peripheral retinal pigment epithelium OU

The *most* likely diagnosis is

a. Usher's syndrome
b. progressive supranuclear palsy (Steele-Richardson-Olszewski syndrome)
c. ocular myasthenia
d. Kearns-Sayre syndrome

N38 Regarding the patient in Question N37, all of the following could be appropriate actions to take at the initial visit *except*

a. perform edrophonium (Tensilon) test
b. schedule muscle biopsy
c. send off mitochondrial genetic analysis
d. schedule cardiac evaluation

N39 A 26-year-old woman presents with progressive visual loss that has occurred over 6 years. Best-corrected visual acuity is 20/80 in each eye. The results of visual field testing are shown in the figure.

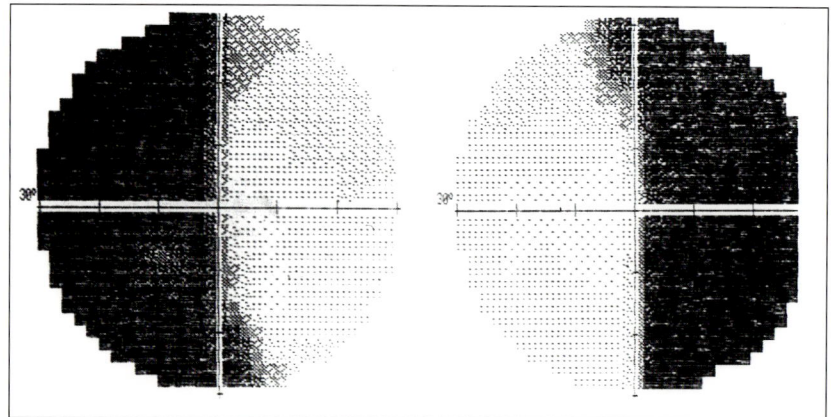

Given the visual fields, which of the following statements is *most* inconsistent with the rest of the evaluation?

a. She has missed a few menstrual cycles over the past year.
b. She is infertile.
c. She has a 3+ to 4+ RAPD OS.
d. She has sparing of the nerve fiber layer along the temporal arcades of both eyes.

N40 A 7-year-old boy is referred by a pediatrician for evaluation of his visual status. The child is said to be slow in school and is being placed in special education. The pediatrician wishes to ensure that a refractive error is not contributing to the poor performance. The child has had three seizures, and a raised papular rash in a butterfly distribution has been noted on his cheeks. Some patchy hypopigmented areas are also seen on the trunk. The child is otherwise well.

The *most* likely diagnosis is

a. tuberous sclerosis (Bourneville's disease)
b. encephalotrigeminal angiomatosis (Sturge-Weber syndrome)
c. juvenile-onset systemic lupus erythematosus with cerebritis
d. neurofibromatosis type I (von Recklinghausen's disease)

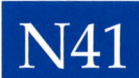

N41 If a fundus abnormality were encountered in the patient in Question N40, which of the following would it *most* likely be?

a. choroidal hemangioma
b. branch retinal artery occlusion
c. retinal astrocytic hamartoma (mulberry astrocytic hamartoma)
d. racemose angioma

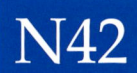

N42 A 30-year-old woman whom you have examined several times in the past for a refractive error consults you as an emergency. In the past, aside from mild myopia, her examinations have always been normal. Specifically, you are sure that there has been no anisocoria or ptosis. The patient complains of a 1-day history of headache and severe pain in the left jaw and left upper neck, with local neck tenderness, and the new onset of ptosis. She tells you that she has taken up karate and had an especially vigorous workout yesterday evening. The results of her examination are as follows:

Best-corrected acuity: 20/20 OU

Pupils: Dim—8 mm OD, 3 mm OS; light—3 mm OD, 2.5 mm OS

Lid fissures: 10 mm OD, 8 mm OS

Motility: Normal

Exophthalmometry: Base 102 mm, OD 18 mm, OS 18 mm

Slit lamp: Normal, no injection of globes

Intraocular pressures: 12 mm Hg OD, 14 mm Hg OS

Fundi: Normal

With this history, the lesion of concern is *most* likely located in the

a. left brain stem
b. left cervical carotid artery
c. left cavernous sinus
d. left orbit

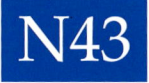

N43 A patient's routine examination is normal except for his pupils. The right pupil is 2.5 mm, the left pupil is 2.0 mm, neither reacts well to light, and both appear to react briskly to near.

Which of the following statements is true?

a. If the patient is a diabetic, no workup is needed.
b. If the fluorescent treponemal antibody (FTA), Lyme titer, and microhemagglutination test (MHA-TP) are positive, the patient should be treated for early Lyme disease, with no spinal tap being performed.
c. If the VDRL is negative, no spinal tap is needed.
d. If the FTA is positive, a spinal tap is needed.

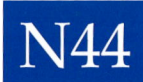

A 23-year-old woman presents with typical optic neuritis OD. She has no history of a prior episode of visual loss in either eye, nor any past history or physical finding to suggest neurologic disease outside of the visual system. The results of the examination are as follows:

Best-corrected acuity: 20/40 OD, 20/20 OS

Ishihara color plates: 6/10 correct OD, 10/10 correct OS

Visual fields: Shown in the figure, parts A and B

The representative MRI is shown in the figure, parts C and D. All images not shown are normal.

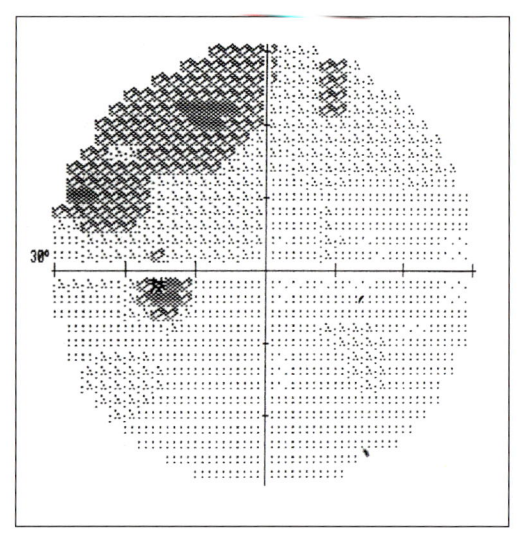

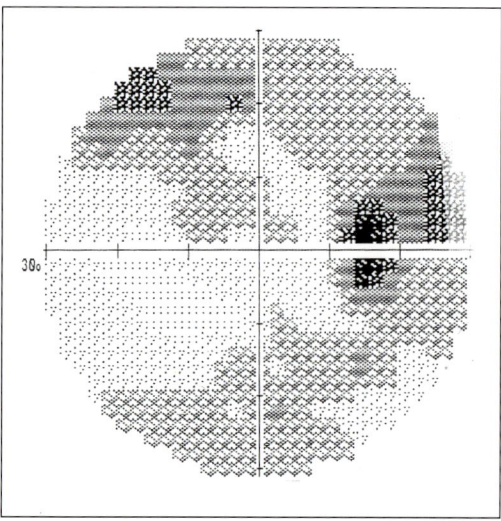

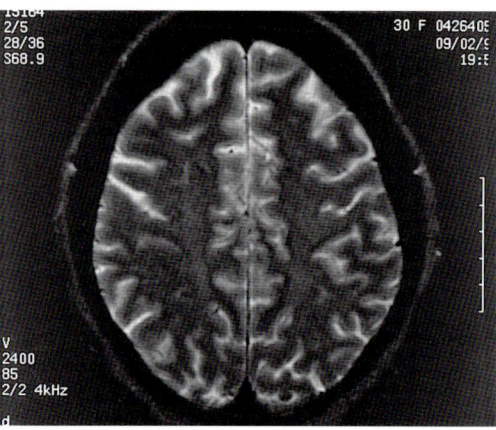

Which of the following statements is true?

a. The patient has the criteria for the diagnosis of multiple sclerosis at this time.
b. The patient may not have had a *prior* optic neuritis OS.
c. The patient should be treated with oral corticosteroids.
d. The patient has at least a 25% chance of developing multiple sclerosis in the next 2 years.

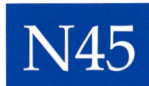

N45 Which of the following findings would be unusual in a patient presenting for an examination before craniotomy for a large pineal tumor?

a. light-near dissociation of the pupils
b. skew deviation
c. convergence-retraction nystagmus only on attempted saccades downward
d. lid retraction

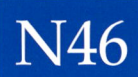

N46 A 37-year-old man's examination is normal, but his history is striking. He has had, in the past few weeks, several bouts of severe right periocular pain associated with the right eye tearing. His nose runs, but only from the right nostril. His wife thinks that the right eye gets red during the episodes of pain. She knows when his pain occurs, because it always awakens him, and thus her, 2 hours before her alarm clock is set to go off.

The *most* likely diagnosis is

a. cluster headache
b. left frontal sinusitis
c. ophthalmoplegic migraine
d. left cervical carotid dissection

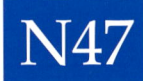

N47 A 16-year-old girl is referred to you for a further opinion. She has had three bouts of orbital pseudotumor. She is well except for what has clinically been diagnosed as asthma. She has had three needle biopsies of the orbit performed. The cytopathologist does not feel that a final diagnosis can be made, as all three demonstrated a mixed polyclonal inflammatory response. She responds to high doses of prednisone, but whenever she is tapered below 20 mg, she seems to flare again with ocular pain and proptosis. In examining her, you notice that the bridge of her nose seems too small for the rest of her nose. She confirms that the bridge is getting smaller, but blames it on the side effects of the prednisone.

Which of the following would be the *least* appropriate next step in her management?

a. Obtain a serum ANCA (antineutrophilic cytoplasmic antibody).
b. Obtain a chest x-ray and urinalysis.
c. Put her on 1 mg/kg of prednisone, do not taper for 1 year, then slowly wean.
d. Perform a biopsy via orbitotomy.

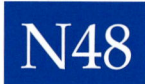

Two patients present with bilateral internuclear ophthalmoplegia. One is 20 years old, and the other is 65. The younger patient has no other medical history, and the 65-year-old has always been well but for recently diagnosed hypertension. Their examinations are otherwise normal.

All of the following statements are true *except*

a. The most likely problem in the younger patient is demyelinating disease.
b. The older patient should be treated with 1 g of methylprednisolone sodium succinate (Solumedrol) daily for 3 days.
c. The older patient probably has a vasculopathic process.
d. The problem in both patients localizes to the pons.

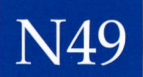

A patient presents with complete bilateral ophthalmoplegia that has lasted 1 week. The lid fissures are 3 mm OU. The pupils are 3 mm OU, round, reactive to light, and without RAPD. The afferent visual system is unaffected, and the patient can read with either eye without difficulty. The patient had a viral episode with diarrhea, nausea, and vomiting 2 days before the onset of the ocular symptoms. Despite having one eye patched, she is ataxic and areflexic. The rest of the examination is normal.

All of the following statements are true *except*

a. The patient probably does not have botulism.
b. The patient should undergo spinal tap.
c. The patient might have Miller Fisher syndrome.
d. The patient probably has myasthenia.

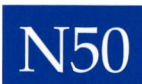

All of the following are true about neuro-ophthalmic disease and childbearing *except*

a. Although pseudotumor cerebri may be seen early in pregnancy, pregnancy may not be a definite risk factor for its development; when seen, pseudotumor cerebri is often self-limited and abates by the fifth month.
b. Preexisting meningiomas do not get worse during pregnancy.
c. Preexisting pituitary tumors may grow during pregnancy and encroach upon the chiasm, causing visual loss, even in the absence of overt apoplexy.
d. Multiple sclerosis may relapse during the postpartum period.

SECTION FIVE

ORBIT AND OPHTHALMIC PLASTIC SURGERY

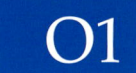

A 10-year-old boy sustained a right upper eyelid laceration after falling from his bicycle. The laceration measures 15 mm and extends from the eyelid margin to above the eyelid crease. There is an avulsed avascular section of the laceration superiorly. The results of his ocular examination are normal except for marked swelling of the eyelid.

The *least* appropriate action in the management of this case is to

a. check the tetanus status
b. repair the eyelid margin
c. discard the avulsed tissue
d. check the status of the levator muscle

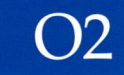

All of the following will prevent a notch of the eyelid margin after a laceration repair *except*

a. reapproximating the tarsus
b. inverting sutures at the eyelid margin
c. everting sutures at the eyelid margin
d. reapproximating the eyelid skin edges

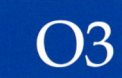

A patient presents with the condition shown in the figure.

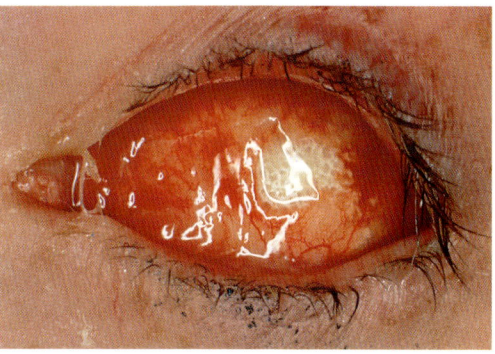

The *least* appropriate treatment for this condition is

a. topical antibiotics
b. scleral patch graft
c. direct closure of the conjunctiva
d. removal of the implant

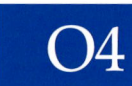

A 27-year-old man presents with the mass shown in the figure. This mass has been present all his life but now is a cosmetic concern for the patient.

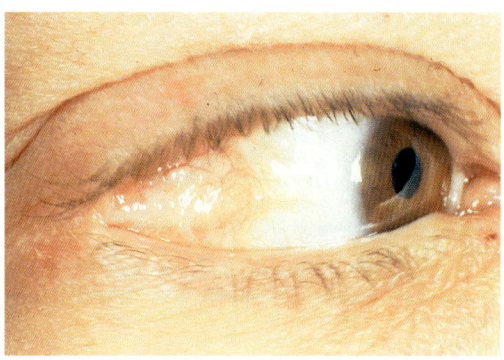

The *most* likely diagnosis is

a. prolapsed lacrimal gland
b. dermolipoma
c. prolapsed orbital fat
d. lymphangioma

The patient in Question O4 desires that his lesion be removed for cosmetic purposes. The *most* appropriate management is

a. fixation in the lacrimal gland fossa
b. laser ablation
c. complete excision
d. partial excision

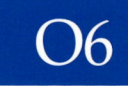

The *least* likely ocular complication from endoscopic sinus surgery is

a. tearing
b. blindness
c. diplopia
d. ptosis

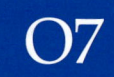

A 56-year-old man complains of an aching sensation around his left eye that has lasted for 6 weeks. The discomfort increases on up gaze. One week ago, he noted blurred vision in the left eye and a low-grade fever. His visual acuity is 20/20 OD and 20/40 OS. The patient has 3 mm of proptosis in the left eye and mild erythema and tenderness around the left eyelid. Results of biomicroscopy and dilated fundus examination are normal.

The *most* helpful diagnostic test for this patient is

a. complete blood count
b. skull films
c. CT scan of the orbits
d. thyroid function tests

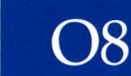 A CT scan of the patient in Question O7 shows clear sinus structures, proptosis, and infiltration of the orbital fat in the left orbit (see the figure).

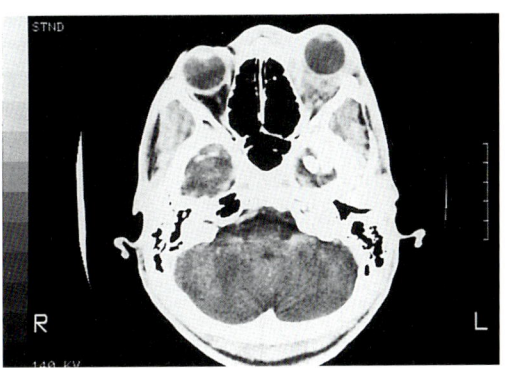

The *most* appropriate initial intervention should include

a. intravenous antibiotics
b. oral corticosteroids
c. orbital irradiation
d. propylthiouracil

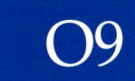 The blood tests of the patient in Question O7 show a normal white blood cell count. The patient has received 48 hours of intravenous antibiotics. The patient's symptoms and signs have not improved. Echography of the orbit fails to show evidence of an orbital abscess. The next therapeutic intervention should include

a. intravenous antibiotics
b. oral corticosteroids
c. orbital irradiation
d. ethmoidectomy

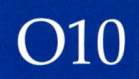 The symptoms of the patient in Question O7 disappear after 48 hours of prednisone 80 mg daily. The *most* likely diagnosis is

a. orbital cellulitis
b. thyroid-related orbitopathy
c. orbital pseudotumor
d. orbital mucocele

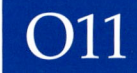 All of the following orbital diseases may improve with corticosteroids *except*

a. orbital lymphoma
b. thyroid-related orbitopathy
c. orbital mucocele
d. orbital pseudotumor

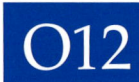

A 75-year-old woman complains of restriction of her upper field of vision and difficulty reading when looking down. She denies any discomfort, epiphora, or diplopia. Her vision is J1+ OU through her well-positioned bifocal segments. A basic tear secretion test is normal. Examination shows an eyelid malposition.

The *most* likely diagnosis is

a. ectropion
b. entropion
c. involutional ptosis
d. dermatochalasis

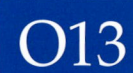

Which of the following is *least* useful in the evaluation of a patient with acquired ptosis?

a. margin-reflex distance
b. interpalpebral fissures
c. levator muscle function
d. frontalis muscle excursion

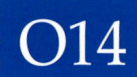

The patient shown in the figure has complained of a droopy left upper eyelid. The results of the eye examination are as follows.

	Right Eye	Left Eye	Normal
Margin-reflex distance	+4 mm	+1.5 mm	+4–5 mm
Levator function	14 mm	15 mm	15 mm
Fissures	10 mm	7.5 mm	10 mm
Eyelid crease	8 mm	12 mm	8–10 mm
Schirmer's test	10 mm	10 mm	

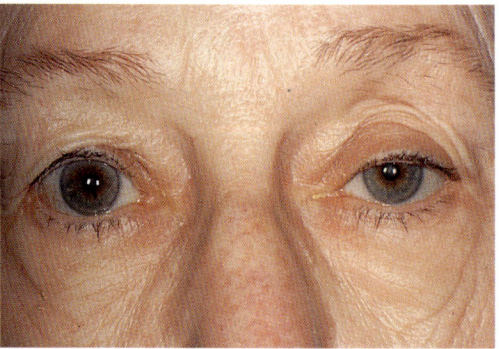

Which of the following is the *most* appropriate surgical management?

a. levator aponeurosis advancement
b. blepharoplasty
c. frontalis suspension
d. levator muscle resection

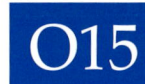

A 7-year-old boy is examined because of bilateral droopy eyelids since birth (see the figure). The visual acuity and ocular motility examinations are normal except for mild limitation of up gaze bilaterally. The eyelid measurements are as follows:

	Right Eye	Left Eye
Margin-reflex distance	0 mm	+0.5 mm
Levator function	3 mm	3 mm
Fissures	5 mm	6 mm
Eyelid crease	absent	absent

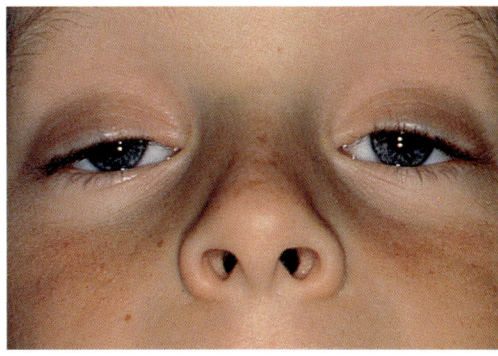

Which of the following is the *most* appropriate surgical management?

a. levator muscle resection
b. frontalis suspension
c. levator aponeurosis advancement
d. Fasanella-Servat procedure

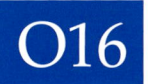

Severe involutional ptosis can be differentiated from severe congenital ptosis by all of the following *except*

a. amount of lid lag in down gaze
b. amount of levator muscle function
c. position of the upper eyelid crease
d. amount of ptosis

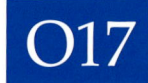 A 32-year-old man has a painless mass located in the superior lateral aspect of the left upper eyelid, which has been present for 4 months. There is no history of trauma, surgery, or chronic conjunctivitis. The results of the ocular examination are normal except for the mobile, translucent mass shown on eversion of the upper eyelid (see the figure).

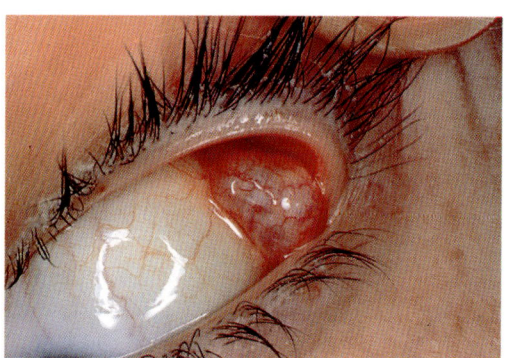

The *most* likely diagnosis is

a. lacrimal ductal cyst
b. lymphoma
c. lipodermoid
d. hematic cyst

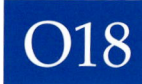 A 55-year-old man reports an 8-month history of a lesion on the medial aspect of the right lower eyelid. The patient had an actinic keratosis removed elsewhere 3 years ago. The ocular examination is unremarkable except for the lesion seen in the figure.

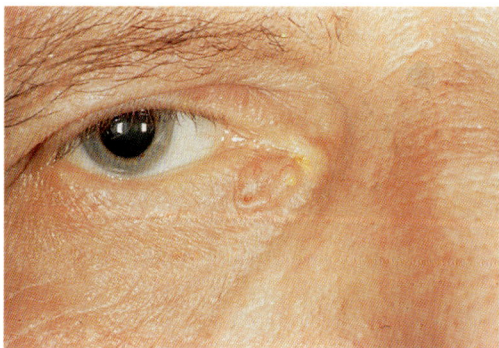

The *most* likely diagnosis is

a. sebaceous cell carcinoma
b. basal cell carcinoma
c. squamous cell carcinoma
d. seborrheic keratosis

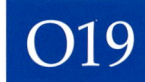 An incisional biopsy is done on the patient in Question O18. The histopathology is shown in the figure.

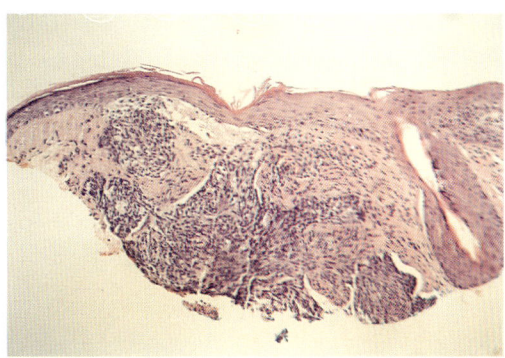

The *most* appropriate management is

a. observation
b. Mohs' surgery
c. radiation
d. liquid nitrogen

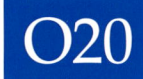 A squamous cell carcinoma of the lower eyelid was excised with controlled margins. The figure shows the resultant defect.

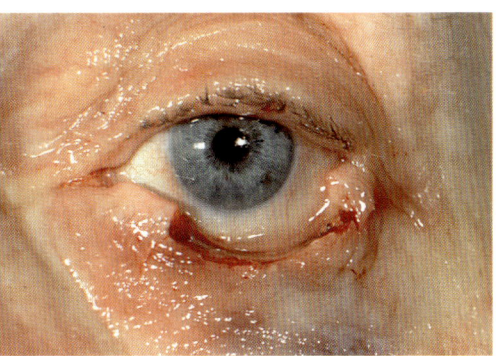

Which of the following is the *most* appropriate management?

a. observation
b. Hughes procedure
c. skin graft
d. Cutler-Beard procedure

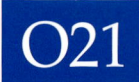 A 68-year-old man complains of irritation and redness of the right eye that has been present for the past 2 months. He has recently been treated for recurrent chalazia and conjunctivitis without relief. The results of visual acuity and anterior and posterior segment examinations are normal. Examination of the regional lymph nodes yields negative results. The right upper eyelid is shown in the figure.

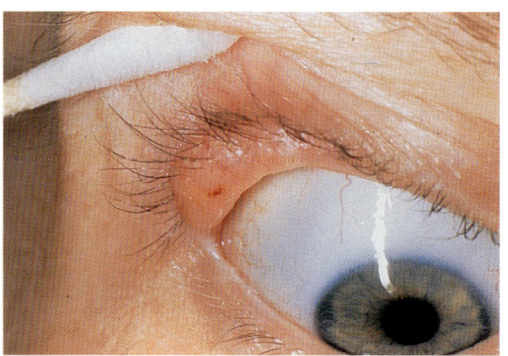

The *most* likely diagnosis is

a. nevus
b. blepharitis
c. sebaceous cell carcinoma
d. viral conjunctivitis

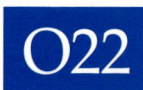 A 37-year-old woman is examined for irritation of the right eye. There is mild conjunctival injection and a follicular reaction. The external examination reveals the lesion shown in the figure.

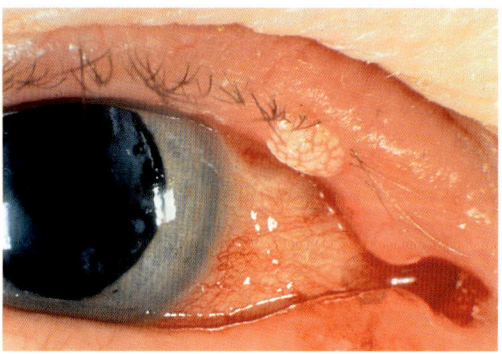

The *most* appropriate management for this patient is

a. excisional biopsy
b. incisional biopsy
c. observation
d. antiviral agents

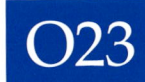 The histopathology of the upper eyelid lesion depicted in Question O22 is shown in the figure.

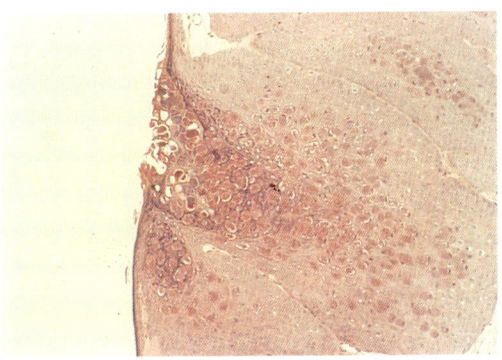

The *most* likely diagnosis is

a. epithelial inclusion cyst
b. keratoacanthoma
c. nevus
d. molluscum contagiosum

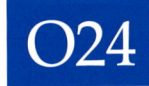 A 75-year-old man presents with the lesion shown in the figure. It has been present for 4 weeks, rapidly increasing in size, and it is painless.

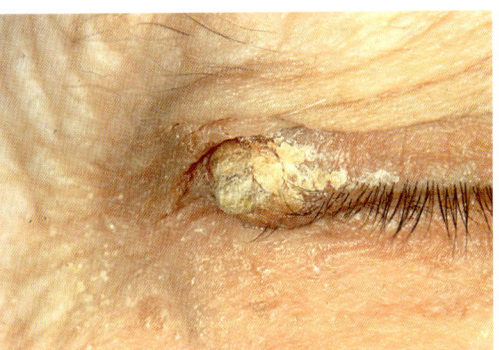

All of the following are characteristics of this lesion *except*

a. malignant potential
b. keratin-filled crater
c. rapid growth
d. spontaneous resolution

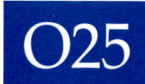 A 47-year-old man with a 1-week history of eye discomfort is evaluated. The patient had an acoustic neuroma resected 3 months ago. The ocular examination shows 5 mm of lagophthalmos, exposure keratopathy, and inferior conjunctival injection. His lower eyelid is shown in the figure.

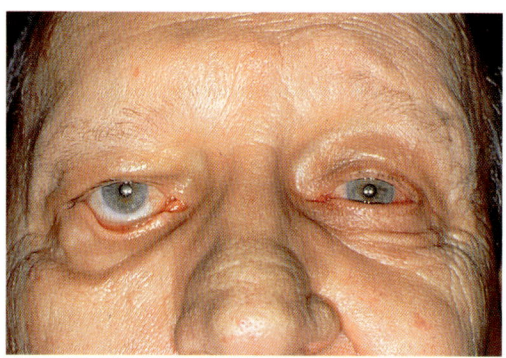

The proper classification for the condition shown is

    a. cicatricial ectropion
    b. paralytic ectropion
    c. involutional ectropion
    d. mechanical ectropion

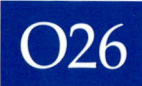 The *least* appropriate management for the patient in Question O25 is

    a. gold weight for the upper eyelid
    b. lid tightening of the lower eyelid
    c. complete tarsorrhaphy
    d. eye lubricants

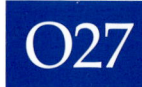 A patient suffered a facial burn 1 year ago, resulting in the eyelid position shown in the figure.

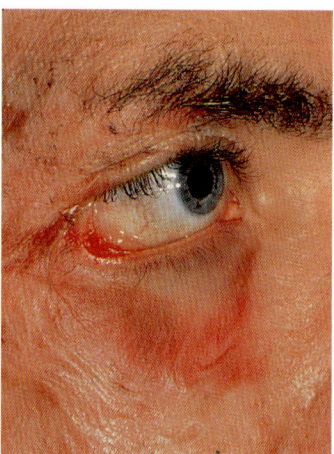

The *least* appropriate long-term management of this condition is

a. split-thickness skin graft
b. full-thickness skin graft
c. lid-tightening procedure
d. release of the cicatrix

O28

A 22-year-old woman is examined for intermittent swelling of the medial canthal lesion shown in the figures. The visual acuity is normal. There is a past history of swelling of this lesion during upper respiratory tract infections.

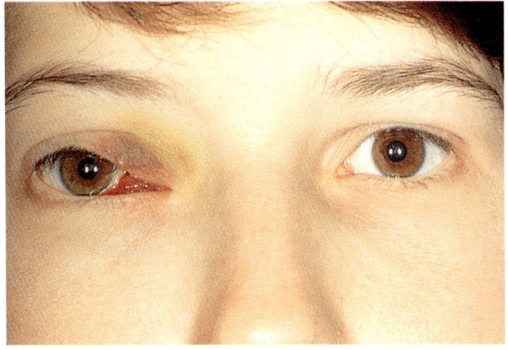
A

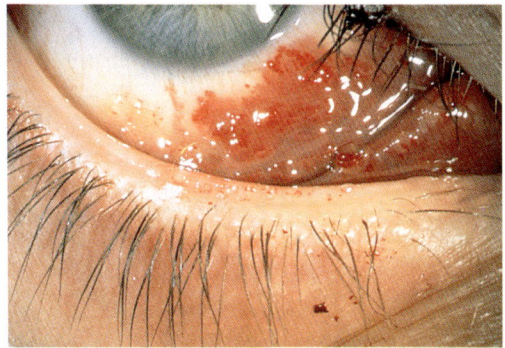
B

The *most* likely diagnosis is

a. lymphoma
b. neurofibroma
c. lymphangioma
d. leukemia

O29

The patient in Question O28 later presents as shown in the figure. The visual acuity is 20/20 OU and the intraocular pressure is 18 mm Hg OU.

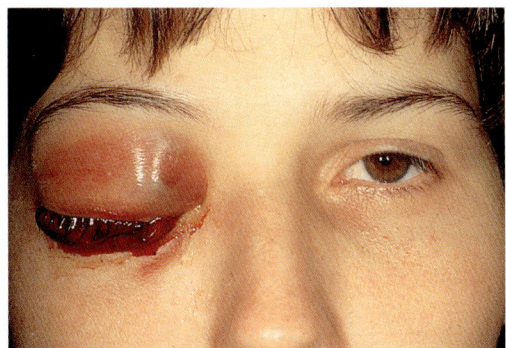

The *most* appropriate management for this patient is

a. biopsy
b. observation
c. chemotherapy
d. radiation

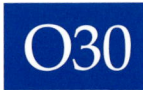 A 54-year-old woman is evaluated for painless bilateral proptosis. Her eyes were normal until 1 year ago. The CT scans are shown in the figures.

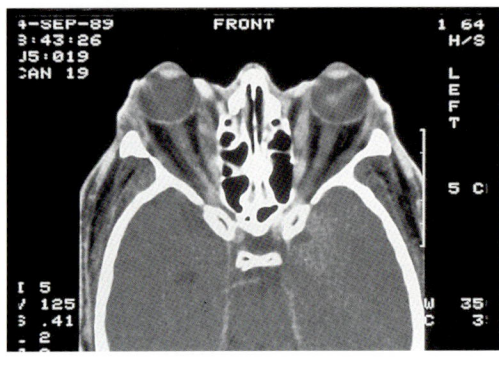
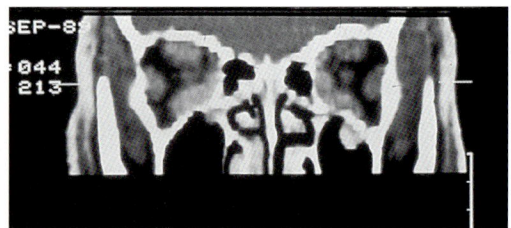

A   B

Which of the eyelid findings listed below is *most* associated with this condition?

a. entropion
b. floppy eyelids
c. ectropion
d. eyelid retraction

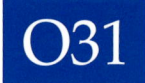 All of the following CT findings are commonly seen with thyroid-related orbitopathy *except*

a. bilateral extraocular muscle involvement
b. sparing of extraocular muscle tendons
c. involvement of extraocular muscle tendons
d. fusiform extraocular muscle involvement

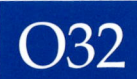 The patient in Question O30 returns 6 months later with decreased vision, worse in the left eye, and a relative afferent pupillary defect. The visual acuity is 20/50 OD and 20/200 OS. The Goldmann visual field of the left eye is shown in the figure.

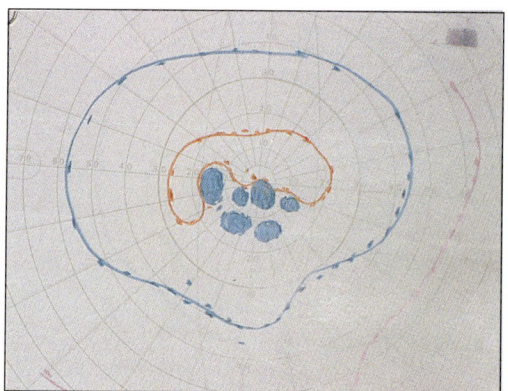

The *most* likely cause for the decreased vision is

a. corneal exposure
b. compressive optic neuropathy
c. refractive error
d. malingering

The *least* appropriate management for the patient in Question O30 is

a. orbital decompression
b. corticosteroids
c. levothyroxine
d. radiation

Which of the following procedures is *least* likely to improve the eyelid position and corneal exposure in the patient shown in the figure?

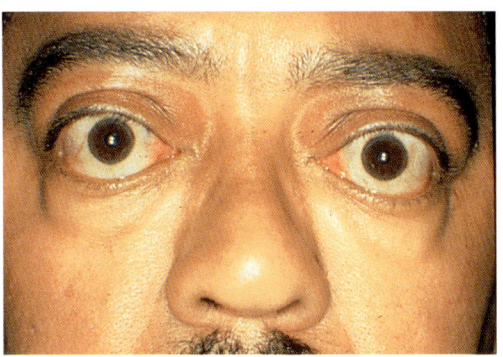

a. lid tightening (lateral tarsal strip)
b. levator recession/müllerectomy
c. lower lid retractor extirpation/spacer graft
d. lateral tarsorrhaphy

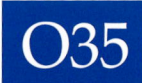 A patient is evaluated for ectropion of his left lower eyelid (see the figure, part A), which is causing epiphora. The ectropion has been present for 1 month. His ocular examination is otherwise normal. The patient's everted eyelid is shown in part B of the figure.

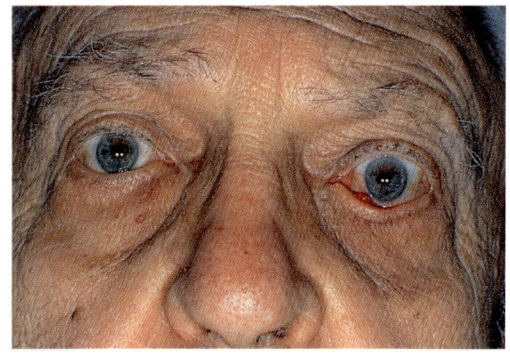
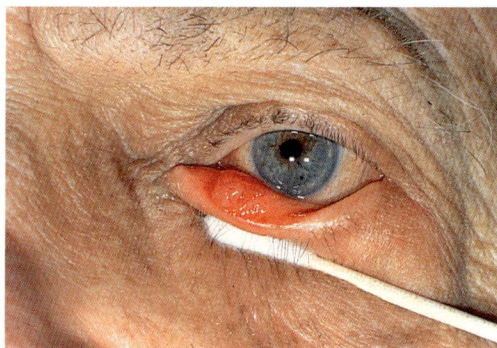

A
B

The *most* likely cause of the ectropion is

a. lymphoma
b. sarcoid
c. Kaposi's sarcoma
d. chalazion

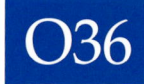 During routine examination of a patient's inferior cul-de-sac, the lesion shown in the figure is observed. The patient is unaware of this lesion and is reportedly in good health. The results of the remainder of the ocular examination are normal.

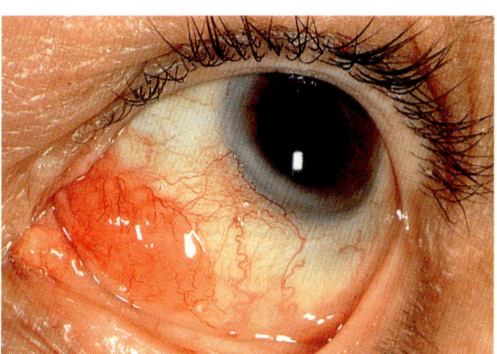

The *most* likely diagnosis is

a. chalazion
b. lymphoproliferative lesion
c. prolapsed orbital fat
d. Kaposi's sarcoma

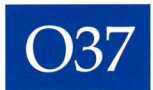 A biopsy is done on the patient in Question O36. The *least* useful test to perform on this biopsy would be

a. culture and sensitivity
b. cell-surface markers
c. permanent sections
d. electron microscopy

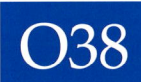 The 7-year-old girl shown in the figure is evaluated for left periorbital discomfort and tenderness that has been present for 24 hours. Her vision is 20/20 OD and 20/60 OS. The left globe is 3 mm proptotic and displaced inferiorly. Pain is present with eye movements. A mild left relative afferent pupillary defect is present. Fundus examination shows choroidal folds superiorly.

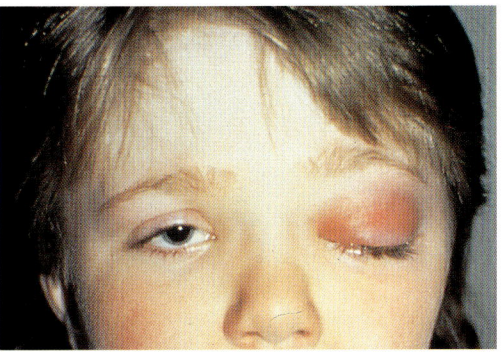

The history and examination are *least* consistent with

a. preseptal cellulitis
b. rhabdomyosarcoma
c. orbital cellulitis
d. pseudotumor

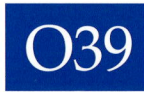

The figures show the CT scans of the patient in Question O38.

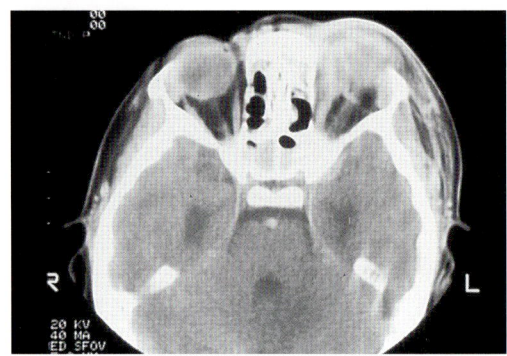
A

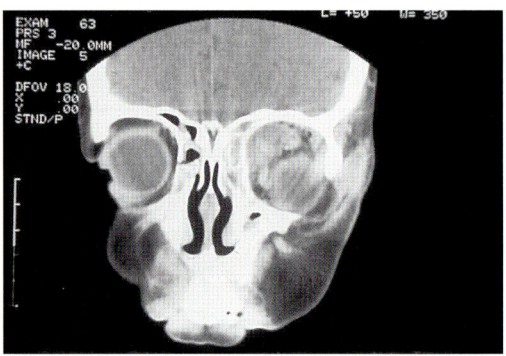
B

The appearance of these scans is *most* consistent with which of the following conditions?

a. orbital abscess
b. rhabdomyosarcoma
c. preseptal cellulitis
d. pseudotumor

You are asked to evaluate a 20-year-old man in the emergency room who has been hit over the left brow with a hockey stick. The visual acuity is 20/20 OD and 20/200 OS. A large hematoma is forming in the left upper eyelid, and the eyelid is tense. A left relative afferent pupillary defect is present. Anterior segment examination reveals a left subconjunctival hemorrhage with a microscopic hyphema. It is not possible to measure the intraocular pressure in the left eye; however, the left globe is tense to digital palpation. Dilated fundus examination of the left eye reveals peripheral retinal edema and pulsation of the central retinal artery.

The *most* appropriate emergent management is to

a. order an emergent CT scan
b. begin intravenous corticosteroids
c. perform a canthotomy and cantholysis
d. perform a paracentesis

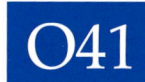 A previously healthy 6-year-old child presents with proptosis of the left eye. Family photographs reveal some prominence of the eye for the past year. One week prior to presentation, the child had a seizure of undetermined cause. Fundus examination reveals choroidal folds OS.

Which one of the following diagnostic tests is *least* useful in this case?

a. MRI
b. CT scan
c. echography
d. fluorescein angiography

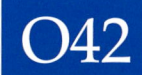 The figures show the MRI results from the patient in Question O41.

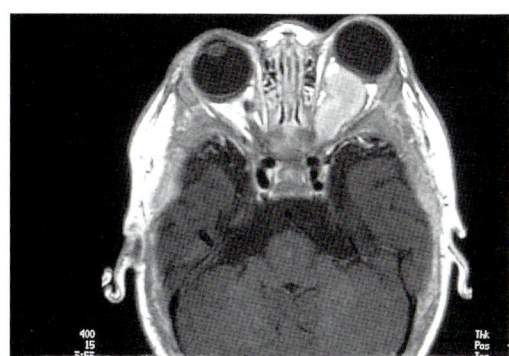
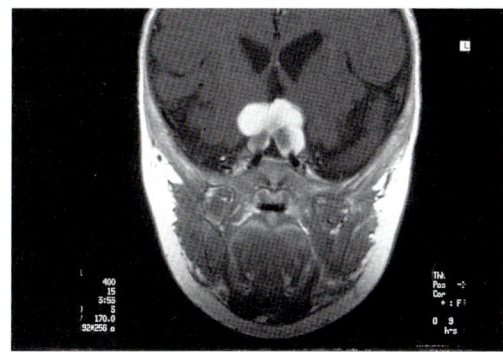

A B

The *most* likely diagnosis is

a. rhabdomyosarcoma
b. optic nerve meningioma
c. optic nerve glioma
d. leukemic infiltration of the optic nerve

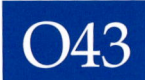 A 55-year-old woman is examined for gradual visual loss in her left eye over 6 months. The visual acuity is 20/20 OD and 20/200 OS. She is found to have 3 mm proptosis and a left relative afferent pupillary defect. Part A of the figure shows the optic nerve head and part B shows the CT scan.

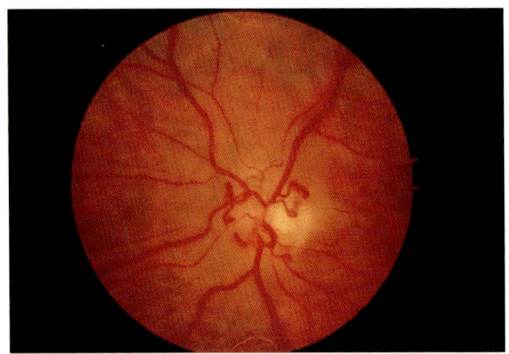
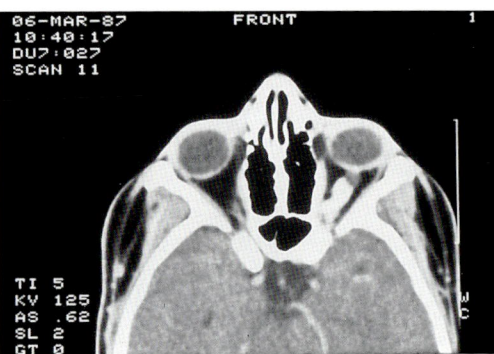

A B

The *least* appropriate management is

a. surgical debulking
b. complete surgical excision
c. radiation following incomplete surgical excision
d. chemotherapy

 Which of the following statements regarding meningiomas is *least* true?

a. Most optic nerve–sparing orbital meningiomas represent extensions of intracranial meningiomas.
b. Meningiomas in children are benign more frequently than meningiomas in adults.
c. Primary meningiomas of the optic nerve occur more frequently in females than in males.
d. Meningiomas occur more frequently in individuals with type 1 neurofibromatosis than in the general population.

 The CT scan of a 61-year-old woman shows diffuse infiltration of the left inferior rectus muscle by metastatic breast carcinoma. All of the following statements about metastatic breast carcinoma to the orbit are true *except*

a. The breast is the most common primary site of metastatic orbital tumors in women.
b. The majority of women have diagnosed breast cancer at the time of orbital involvement.
c. Metastases to the choroid are more common than metastases to the orbit.
d. Enophthalmos is more common than proptosis in this condition.

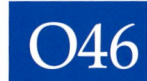 Potential advantages of MRI over CT scanning include all of the following *except*

a. MRI does not expose the patient to radiation.
b. MRI allows for better evaluation of lesions that extend from the orbit to the cranium.
c. MRI is unaffected by motion artifact.
d. MRI can generate high-quality axial, coronal, and sagittal images without repositioning the patient.

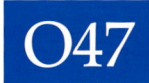 A 38-year-old woman presents with proptosis of her left eye. She complains of periodic headaches, especially in the brow area. On examination, her left eye is noted to be displaced inferiorly and laterally. The figures show the CT scans.

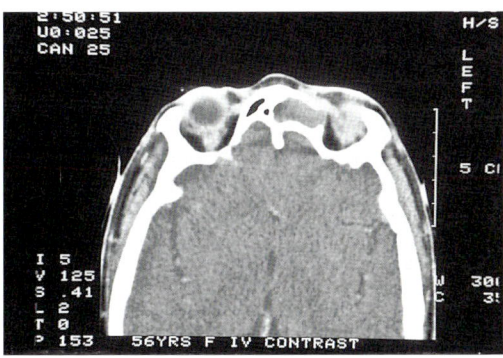
A

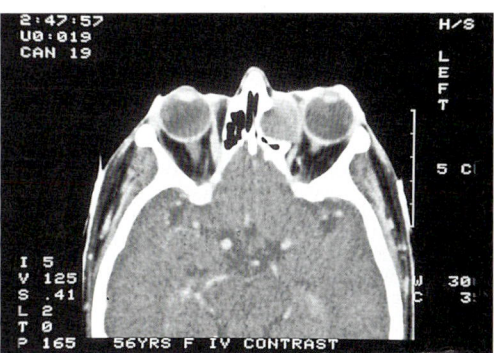
B

The *most* likely diagnosis is

a. lymphangioma
b. lymphoma
c. orbital abscess
d. mucocele

 The *most* appropriate management of the patient in Question O47 is

a. observation
b. nasal decongestants and prophylactic oral antibiotics
c. drainage via percutaneous needle aspiration
d. surgical resection

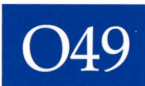 A 17-year-old boy is evaluated for a 2-day history of painful swelling of the right upper eyelid. The swelling began 24 hours after a wrestling tournament. The patient is healthy, with no history of past ocular problems. On examination the vision is 20/20 in each eye. Abduction of the right eye is limited and associated with pain. Moderate injection of the right temporal bulbar conjunctiva is present. The CT scans are shown in the figures.

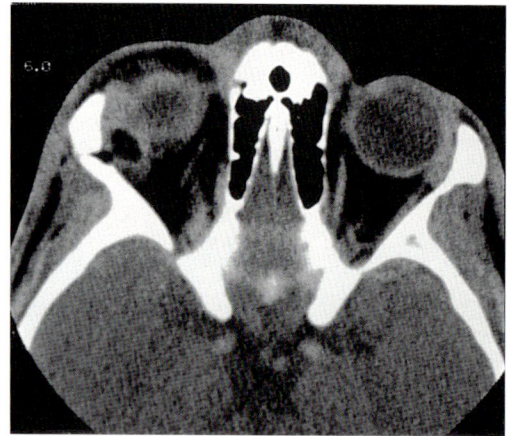

A

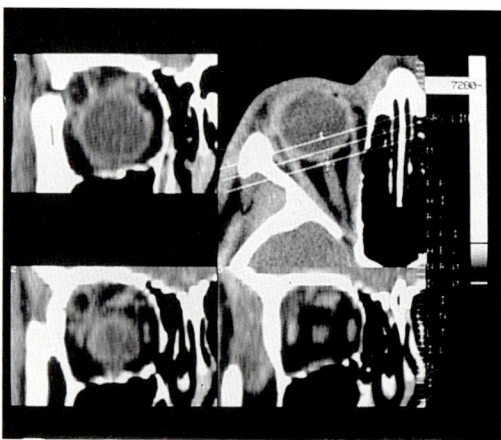

B

The *most* likely diagnosis is

a. fracture of the lateral wall of the orbit
b. orbital cellulitis
c. preseptal cellulitis
d. ruptured dermoid cyst

 The *most* appropriate treatment for the patient in Question O49 is

a. intravenous antibiotics
b. oral prednisone
c. surgical excision
d. warm compresses

SECTION SIX
PEDIATRIC OPHTHALMOLOGY AND STRABISMUS

P1 A day-care worker has given birth to an infant with severe unilateral microphthalmia (see the figure) and a cataract. The mother reports possible exposure to chickenpox during her pregnancy.

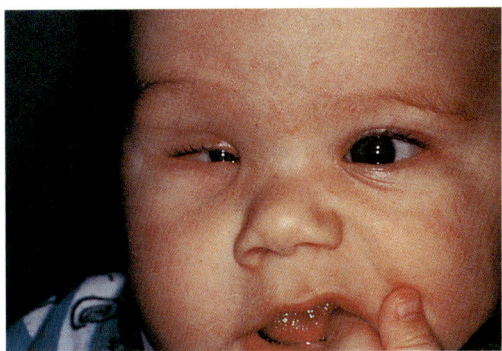

Which of the following ocular abnormalities is least consistent with the diagnosis of an intrauterine varicella infection?

a. cataract
b. chorioretinitis
c. Horner's syndrome
d. aniridia

P2 You are asked to evaluate in the newborn nursery a low-birth-weight infant with possible eye anomalies. During your examination, you instruct the nursing personnel to dilate the child's eyes with a mixture of 0.5% cyclopentolate and 2.5% phenylephrine ophthalmic solution.

All of the following additional instructions should be given to the nursing personnel *except*

a. Delay the infant's feeding for at least 2 hours.
b. Temporarily occlude the nasolacrimal puncta after administering the drops.
c. Administer or increase supplemental oxygen.
d. Closely observe the vital signs.

P3 A 4-month-old infant girl is noted by her parents to have the unusual appearance of her right eye shown in the figure, part A. The otherwise healthy child was born 3 weeks prematurely with a birth weight of 5 pounds 6 ounces. Your examination reveals a normal left eye. The right eye demonstrates shallowing of the anterior chamber and a clear crystalline lens, as well as the retrolental and retinal abnormalities shown in the figures. Examinations of the parents and an older sibling are unremarkable.

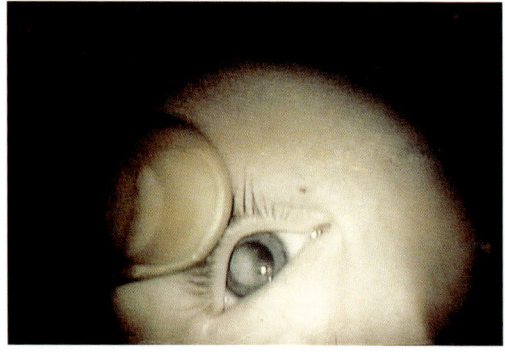
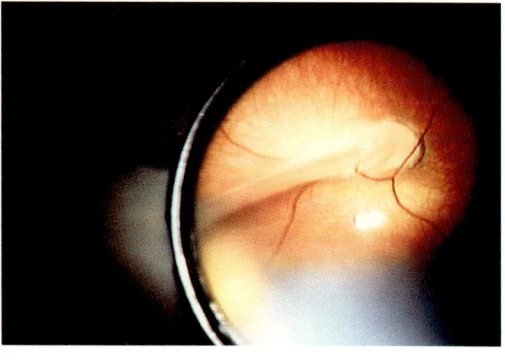

A
B

The *most* likely diagnosis is

a. persistent hyperplastic primary vitreous
b. Norrie's disease
c. incontinentia pigmenti
d. familial exudative vitreoretinopathy

P4 A 4-month-old infant boy presents with epiphora of the right eye that has been present since shortly after birth. Mucoid discharge can be expressed from the puncta with external pressure over the right nasolacrimal sac. The *most* reasonable treatment would be

a. observation
b. massage of the nasolacrimal sac
c. probing of the nasolacrimal duct
d. irrigation of the nasolacrimal duct

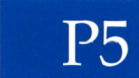

A 6-month-old infant boy demonstrates the ocular deviation shown in the figure. Each eye is able to abduct normally. The child was born after a normal, full-term pregnancy by a normal delivery.

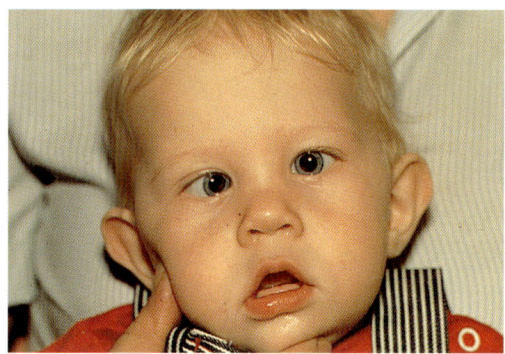

Considering the most likely diagnosis, all of the following statements about this condition are true *except*

a. Amblyopia is commonly associated.
b. Abduction and adduction movements are often asymmetric.
c. Vertical deviations are commonly associated.
d. Patients with this condition rarely require glasses during childhood.

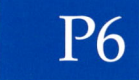

A 2-week-old infant boy presents with the ocular findings shown in the figure. There is no history of ocular trauma or inflammation.

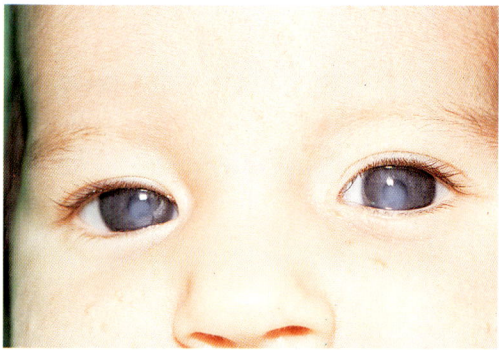

All of the following statements are true *except*

a. Glaucoma is commonly associated with this condition.
b. This condition is usually bilateral.
c. Systemic abnormalities are rare.
d. This condition may have been caused by neural crest dysgenesis.

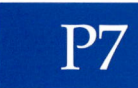 A 3-month-old infant presents with nystagmus and poor fixation responses. The undilated anterior segment findings, which are similar in both eyes, are shown in the figure. The posterior segment reveals small optic discs and indistinct foveae.

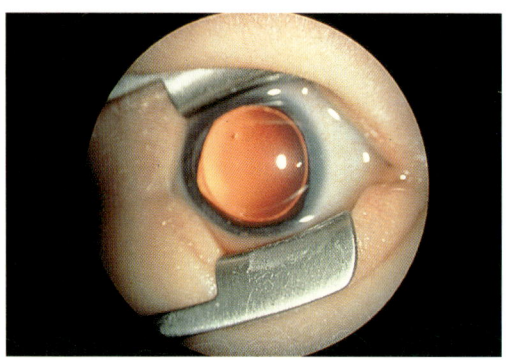

What is the next *most* important step in managing this patient?

a. Obtain a family history.
b. Monitor for amblyopia.
c. Treat with tinted contact lenses.
d. Evaluate for Wilms' tumor.

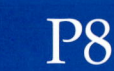 The 3-year-old child shown in the figure received surgery for esotropia at age 1 year. His parents are unhappy with his appearance of upturned eyes. In primary gaze, there is an 8-prism-diopter esotropia. A V pattern is present, with a difference in the deviation from down gaze to up gaze of 15 prism diopters. Under a cover, each eye has a very noticeable hyperdeviation but there is no corresponding hypodeviation on alternate-cover testing. On examination, you demonstrate elevation of each eye in adduction, a right hypertropia on left gaze, and a left hypertropia on right gaze.

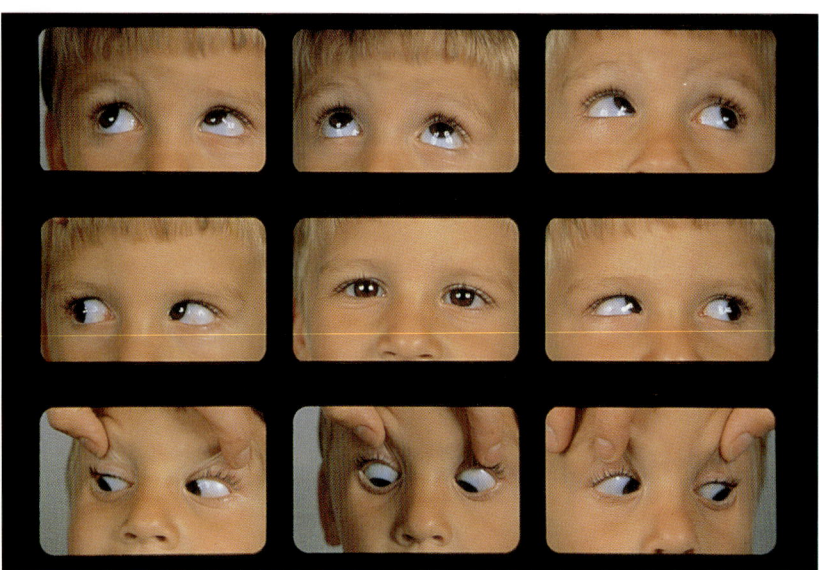

The *most* reasonable operation for this child would be

a. bilateral inferior oblique myectomy
b. bilateral superior rectus recession
c. bilateral inferior oblique recession with anterior displacement
d. bilateral inferior oblique and superior rectus recession

P9 A 2-year-old child has been referred for wandering of one eye that has been evident for the past few months. Using binocular fixation-pattern techniques, you detect reduced vision in that eye. The anterior segment is normal, but the optic nerve is as shown in the figure. The posterior segment of the other eye is normal.

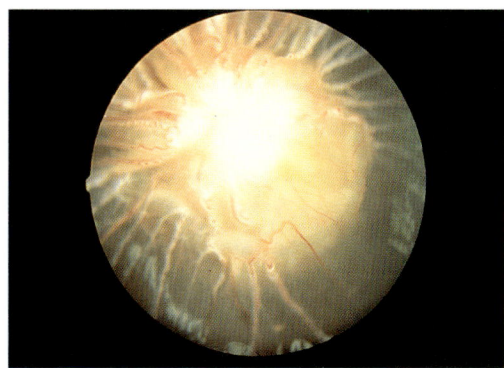

Which of the following statements about the condition shown is true?

a. Visual acuity in the affected eye is usually better than 20/200.
b. The condition is associated with seizures and early death.
c. The condition is hereditary.
d. Retinal detachments are associated with this condition.

P10 An otherwise healthy, 3-week-old newborn presents with bilateral conjunctivitis (see the figure).

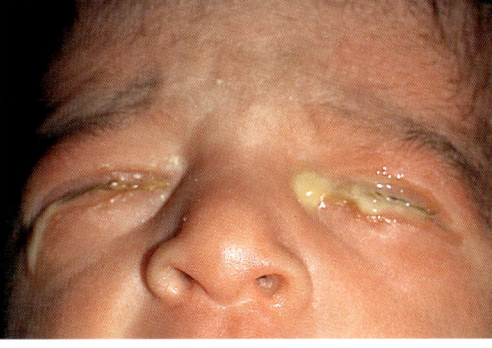

How would you initiate management?

a. Start broad-spectrum systemic antibiotics.
b. Start broad-spectrum topical antibiotics.
c. Obtain conjunctival specimens for microbiology.
d. Obtain blood cultures.

P11 All of the following statements about chlamydial conjunctivitis of the newborn are true *except*

a. It is the most common infectious cause of neonatal conjunctivitis.
b. It is commonly associated with pneumonitis.
c. Oral erythromycin should be prescribed.
d. Silver nitrate 1% solution provides prophylaxis.

P12 A mother complains that her 6-year-old daughter has had increased wandering of her left eye over the past year. Your examination notes an intermittent exotropia of 35 prism diopters with fixation at distance and 5 prism diopters of exophoria with fixation at near. Her uncorrected visual acuity is 20/20 OD and 20/20 OS. After a discussion with the mother, you decide on surgical treatment.

Which of the following tests would be *least* helpful in surgical management of this patient?

a. 30-minute occlusion test
b. +3.00 lens test
c. cycloplegic refraction
d. Worth four-dot test

P13 A 7-year-old boy complains of decreased vision in the right eye. The child also has lymphadenopathy, malaise, and a low-grade fever. On examination, the best-corrected visual acuity is counting fingers OD and 20/20 OS. The left fundus is normal; the right fundus is shown in the figure.

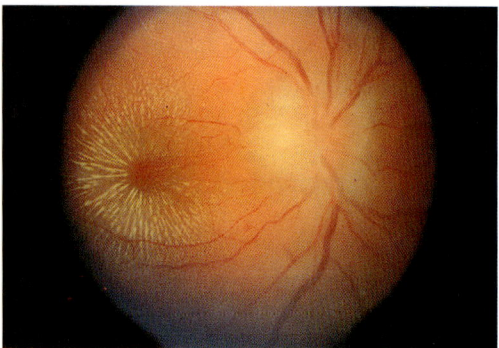

All of the following diseases are consistent with the clinical picture *except*

a. multiple sclerosis
b. Lyme disease
c. syphilis
d. cat-scratch disease

P14 A 4-month-old boy is brought in for evaluation because of visual inattention and nystagmus. His pupils do not respond to light and he has a refractive error of +4.00 OU. Both fundi appear normal.

The *most* likely diagnosis is

a. Leber's optic neuropathy
b. cortical blindness
c. X-linked congenital stationary night blindness
d. Leber's congenital amaurosis

P15 A 6-month-old child is brought in for evaluation of nystagmus and decreased vision. His optic discs are shown in the figure.

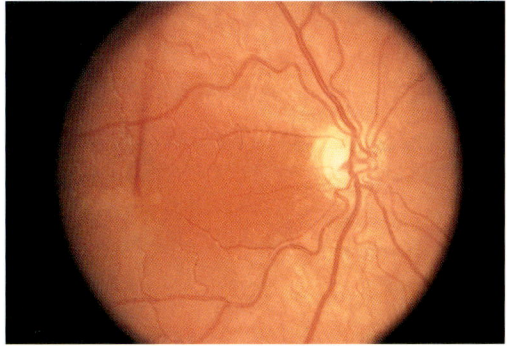
A

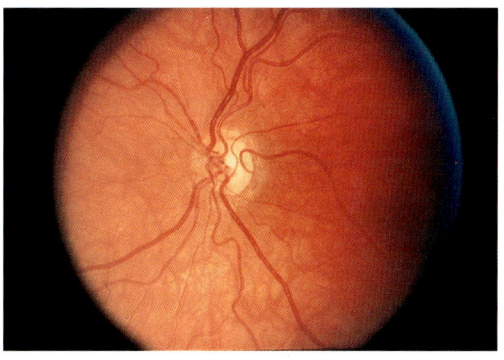
B

Which of the following is the *least* important consideration in managing this patient?

a. inheritance pattern
b. pituitary hormonal dysfunction
c. association with brain anomalies
d. visual development

P16 A 5-year-old child with horizontal nystagmus sees 20/50 when her head is held straight but can see 20/25 by adopting a 45° left head turn. The nystagmus is unchanged when fixing on a near target.

Which surgical approach would be *most* likely to reduce her head turn?

a. Recess the right medial rectus and the left lateral rectus muscles. Resect the right lateral rectus and the left medial rectus muscles.
b. Recess both medial rectus muscles and resect both lateral rectus muscles.
c. Recess the left medial rectus and the right lateral rectus muscles. Resect the left lateral rectus and the right medial rectus muscles.
d. Recess the left medial rectus muscle and resect the left lateral rectus muscle.

P17 The child shown in the figure has had ptosis of the right upper eyelid since birth. When asked to fixate on a distant or near target, she demonstrates a chin-up head position. The alternate-cover test is normal. The induced prism test reveals a preference for the left eye, suggesting decreased vision in her right eye.

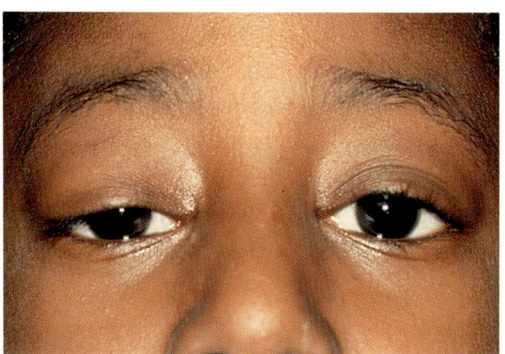

The *most* likely cause of her reduced vision is

a. anisometropic amblyopia
b. deprivation amblyopia
c. strabismic amblyopia
d. chorioretinal coloboma

P18 A 2-year-old boy presents with a history of crossing of his left eye that has been noted by his parents over the past 3 months. Examination reveals a dense total cataract in the left eye. The anterior segment is otherwise normal. The right eye is normal. Both pupils react normally. The past medical history is unremarkable. The next step should be

a. ocular ultrasound
b. urinalysis for reducing substances
c. observation
d. cataract extraction

P19 You are asked to see a 6-month-old infant for suspected shaken baby syndrome. Assuming that the child was abused, what ocular abnormality are you *most* likely to find?

a. subconjunctival hemorrhage
b. retinal hemorrhage
c. iris sphincter tear
d. retinal fold

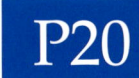

With regard to the patient in Question P19, which of the following statements is true?

a. Retinal hemorrhages associated with child abuse usually occur without intracranial hemorrhage.
b. Timing of the alleged abuse can be estimated by characteristics of the retinal hemorrhages.
c. Retinal hemorrhages in children can result from cardiopulmonary resuscitation.
d. Children diagnosed with shaken baby syndrome have a low incidence of permanent neurologic deficits.

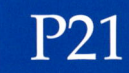

A 3-year-old child was found by his pediatrician to have possible decreased acuity in one eye. Evaluation by an ophthalmologist using the illiterate E test demonstrated a visual acuity of 20/25 OD and 20/60 OS. Cycloplegic retinoscopy revealed mild hyperopia OD but an irregular streak OS that appears hyperopic in the lens periphery but myopic centrally. After a period of observation, the patient showed reduced acuity OS secondary to a lens opacity (see the figure).

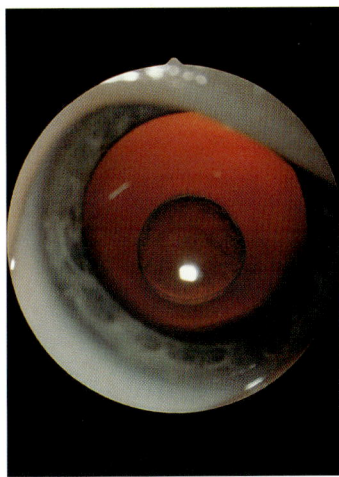

This type of cataract is typically associated with

a. poor visual acuity outcome after surgery
b. progressive involvement of the fellow eye
c. an otherwise anatomically normal eye
d. galactosemia

P22 A 3-year-old girl is referred by her pediatrician for ophthalmologic evaluation. She has had a recent episode of painful swelling of the right knee. Several months prior to that she had swelling of the left elbow. Which of the following statements is true?

a. Ocular involvement is unlikely because more than one joint is affected.
b. Initial ocular signs usually include conjunctival injection.
c. A positive antinuclear antibody (ANA) implies significant ocular risk.
d. If the patient has no ocular manifestations after 3 years, further ophthalmologic follow-up is usually unnecessary.

P23 The patient in Question P22 develops chronic anterior uveitis. In this case, all of the following statements are true *except*

a. The patient is also at risk for developing cataract, band keratopathy, and posterior synechiae.
b. If a cataract develops in this condition, visual acuity outcome is usually poor.
c. Visual prognosis is worse if the uveitis precedes the systemic condition.
d. Glaucoma is usually secondary to a pupillary-block mechanism.

P24 A child is referred for evaluation of an "abnormal pupil." The pupillary appearance is shown in the figure.

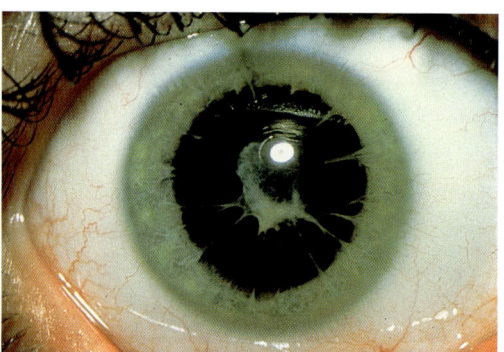

This finding

a. is likely to lead to lens opacification
b. demonstrates a growth that should be surgically removed
c. represents failed regression of the primary vitreous
d. is compatible with good visual acuity

P25 An infant in the newborn nursery is found to have bilateral lens opacities of the type shown in the figure.

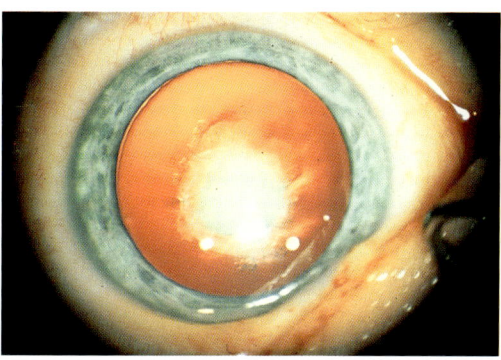

All of the following are true about this condition *except*

a. Evaluation for systemic disease is not indicated.
b. Corneal diameter is usually small.
c. A family history of congenital cataracts is common.
d. The risk of glaucoma after cataract surgery is low.

P26 A 16-year-old boy has a history of normal vision in both eyes. He presents complaining of a sudden decrease in vision in the right eye. His visual acuity is 20/200 OD and 20/15 OS. A relative afferent pupillary defect is present in the right eye, and confrontation visual fields reveal a dense central scotoma OD. Fundus examination reveals a normal macula with a hyperemic-appearing disc OD. The result of MRI of the head and optic nerves is normal.

If an abnormality in this patient's DNA related to visual loss were found, it would *most* likely reveal

a. a mutation in the rhodopsin gene on chromosome 3
b. a mutation on the X chromosome
c. a mutation of the mitochondrial DNA
d. chromosome 13 deletion

P27 A 6-year-old boy was noted to have abnormal vision on a school screening. The ophthalmologist finds his visual acuity to be 20/100 OD and 20/20 OS. When tested with a neutral-density filter, his acuity is 20/60 OD and 20/30 OS. He has a very small esotropia and a refractive error of +1.75 sphere OD and +1.00 sphere OS. He is treated with occlusion therapy of the left eye for 50% of his waking hours. After 3 months, his visual acuity is 20/80 OD and 20/20 OS.

What is the *most* likely reason for his poor response to treatment?

a. inadequate occlusion therapy
b. incomplete treatment of refractive error
c. irreversible functional amblyopia
d. subtle organic abnormality of the macula or optic nerve

P28 Of the following case scenarios, which is the *least* likely to show visual improvement (≥20/40) with full-time occlusion therapy?

a. a 4-year-old child with esotropia of unknown duration whose visual acuity is 20/25 OD and 20/200 OS
b. an 8-year-old child with a refraction of +3.50 OD and +1.00 OS whose best-corrected visual acuity is 20/200 OD and 20/25 OS
c. a 2-year-old child following surgery and contact lens fitting for a unilateral traumatic cataract of 4 months' duration
d. a 2-year-old child found on routine examination to have an anomalous optic nerve head OD and who demonstrates poor fixation and following movements with that eye

P29 You are asked to examine a premature infant with bronchopulmonary dysplasia who is receiving supplemental oxygen by nasal cannula. You note the presence of 4 clock hours of stage 2, zone II retinopathy of prematurity (ROP) in the right eye and 2 clock hours of stage 1, zone II ROP in the left eye. The neonatologist would like your opinion on the level of oxygen to administer. Which one of the following approaches would you recommend?

a. Increase supplemental oxygen to maintain PaO_2 of 98%.
b. Decrease supplemental oxygen until ROP demonstrates regression.
c. Make no change in the supplemental oxygen.
d. Do not rely on the ocular condition in determining oxygen requirements.

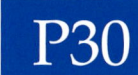

A 3-month-old infant has a history of a difficult birth with prolonged hypoxia. The child is noted to have severe neurologic impairment, including poor visual response. The ocular examination demonstrates no apparent visual fixation responses. Wandering ocular movements are present but are not typical of nystagmus. The remainder of the examination, including assessment of the pupils, retina, and optic nerve, appears normal.

Which of the following is the *best* method for predicting the visual outcome?

a. visual evoked responses
b. CT scan
c. electroretinogram
d. following the patient with sequential examinations

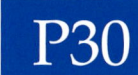

A 38-year-old man was accidentally struck in the right eye with a bungee cord one day prior to your examination. The patient complains of double vision, especially when looking down. He has noticed no change in the vision in his right eye. There is a small laceration of the inferior conjunctiva. Ocular motility is shown in the figure. Forced-duction testing demonstrates slight restriction to elevation and depression. There is 1 mm of proptosis of the right eye. A CT scan of the orbit reveals soft-tissue swelling but no fracture.

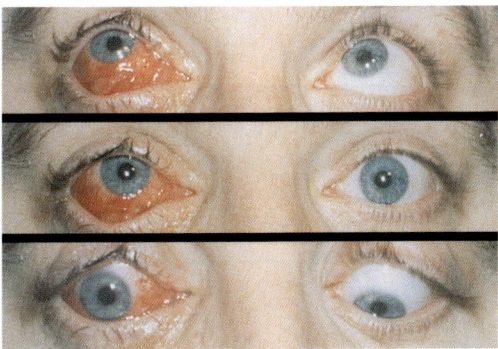

What is the *most* likely cause for his ocular motility abnormality?

a. blowout fracture of the orbital floor
b. inferior rectus paresis
c. traumatic Brown's syndrome
d. laceration of the inferior rectus muscle

P32 A 27-year-old woman initially presents to you with a history of head injury 3 days previously in an automobile accident. The patient complains of constant double vision. The ocular versions are shown in the figure. The remainder of the examination is normal.

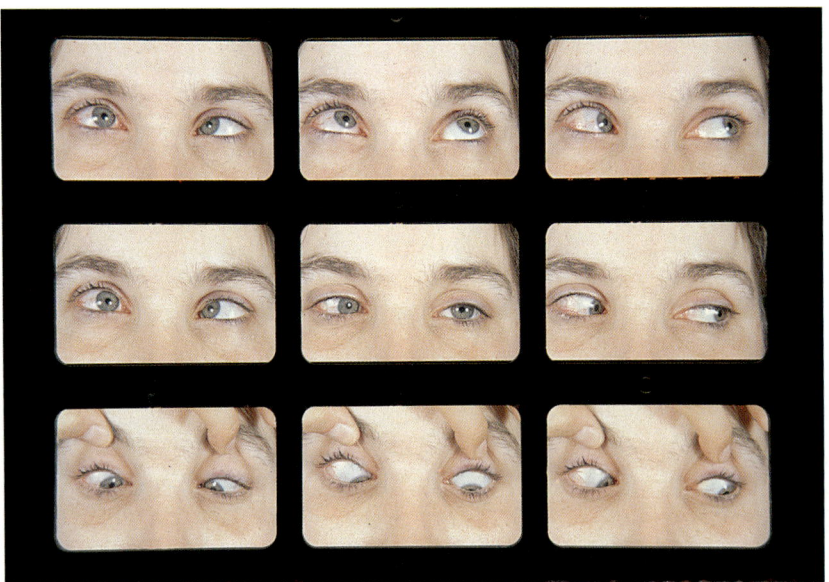

The *best* treatment option at this time would be

a. occlusion of the left eye and reevaluation in 1 to 2 weeks
b. botulinum toxin injection of the right medial rectus muscle
c. recession and resection procedure in the right eye
d. occlusion of the right eye and observation

P33 Cytomegalovirus (CMV) is the most common intrauterine infection and has been isolated from the urine in up to 3% of newborns. A small percentage of these infants show clinical symptoms in the neonatal period and have widespread congenital anomalies. All of the following are typical congenital anomalies associated with intrauterine CMV infection *except*

a. hepatosplenomegaly
b. chorioretinitis
c. limb anomalies
d. microphthalmia

P34 A 30-year-old male accountant sustained a head injury as a result of an automobile accident 8 months previously. This patient's chief complaint is double vision when reading. There is no deviation in primary gaze, but a 15-prism-diopter esotropia is present in down gaze. There is a left hypertropia of 8 prism diopters in right gaze and a right hypertropia of 10 prism diopters in left gaze. Excyclotorsion of 6° is present in primary gaze, increasing to 15° in down gaze. Ocular versions demonstrate underaction of both superior oblique muscles.

What is the *best* treatment option for this patient?

a. reading glasses with prisms
b. bilateral superior oblique tucks
c. bilateral inferior oblique weakening procedures
d. advancement of the anterior fibers of both superior oblique muscles

P35 An 18-month-old child presents with a 6-month history of crossing of the left eye and a 6-week history of a white pupil in the same eye. The physical examination reveals a complete and diffuse haze in the vitreous. No retinal detail can be discerned. There is a suggestion of a mass lesion behind the haze. The CT scan is shown in the figure.

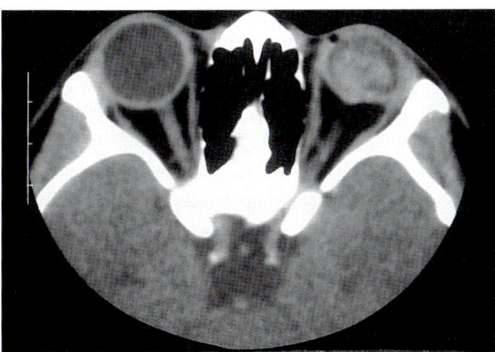

Appropriate management steps might include all of the following *except*

a. ultrasound
b. titer for toxocariasis
c. titer for toxoplasmosis
d. vitreous tap and histopathologic diagnosis

P36 All of the following are true about children with heritable retinoblastoma *except*

a. They may have a visible deletion at chromosome 13q14.
b. They may be unilaterally affected.
c. The majority have no family history.
d. Heritable and nonheritable retinoblastoma have an equal risk of secondary cancers.

P37 A 2-year-old boy presents with emesis, weight loss, and decreased appetite of 2 weeks' duration. The child has a history of retinoblastoma that required enucleation of the right eye and radiation of the left eye. He has been followed every 3 months by examination under anesthesia with no evidence of new or recurrent retinal tumors. A CT scan with contrast is obtained (see the figure).

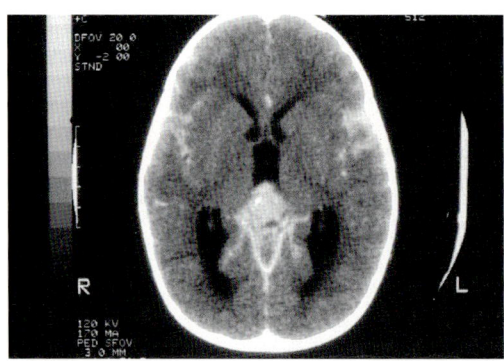

The findings on the scan are *most* likely

a. metastatic retinoblastoma
b. pineal blastoma
c. metastatic neuroblastoma
d. osteosarcoma

P38 A 3-year-old girl presents to your office with wandering of the left eye that has been present for the past 3 months. Examination reveals 3 mm of proptosis of the left eye, a left relative afferent pupillary defect, and optic atrophy OS. Multiple skin lesions are noted on the child's body, as shown in the figure, part A. MRI is obtained, as shown in the figure, part B.

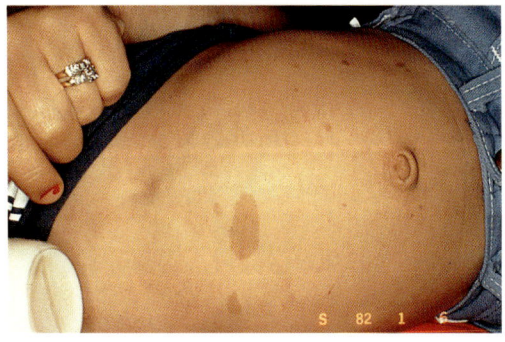
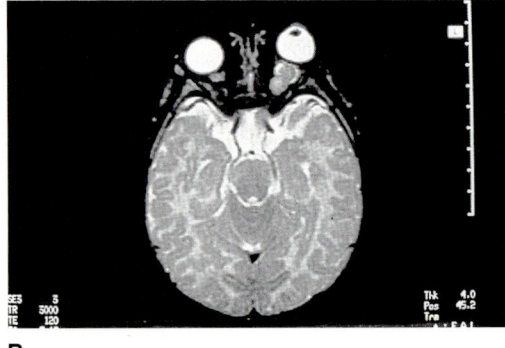

A   B

All of the following are true in this case *except*

a. In older patients, Lisch nodules are usually present.
b. The lesion present on the MRI is usually more aggressive in children than in adults.
c. Associated reactive meningeal hyperplasia may cause a biopsy to be misdiagnosed as meningioma.
d. Histologically, the lesion is a low-grade astrocytoma.

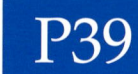

P39 A 20-year-old man has undergone a 4 mm right medial rectus recession for acquired esotropia. Shortly after surgery he developed exotropia and diplopia. The motility examination reveals a widened eyelid fissure with limited adduction of the operated eye. Cover testing shows exotropia in primary gaze that increases on left gaze (see the figure). The remainder of the ocular examination is normal.

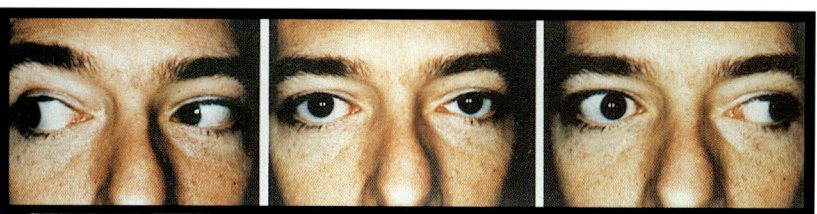

The *most* likely diagnosis is

a. partial third-nerve paresis
b. slipped medial rectus muscle
c. postoperative restriction
d. sensory exotropia

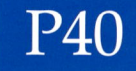

P40 A pediatrician calls to refer a 3-year-old Caucasian boy with a 1-week history of esotropia, abduction limitation, and face turn. There is no history of ocular disease or surgery. The patient is brought in for examination 3 days after the initial phone consultation. The parents have noted a slight improvement in the crossed eyes. The child has no history of trauma but did have a flu-like illness 1 week prior to onset of the esotropia. The ocular examination is normal.

Your workup at this time might include all of the following *except*

a. neurology referral
b. MRI
c. observation
d. erythrocyte sedimentation rate

P41 A 5-year-old boy who had allogenic bone marrow transplantation 1 year ago for acute lymphocytic leukemia presents for routine eye examination. All of the following are ocular complications of bone marrow transplantation *except*

a. cataract
b. superficial punctate keratopathy
c. iris heterochromia
d. retinal hemorrhage

P42 A 13-year-old boy presents with a 6-month history of headaches, blurred vision, and intermittent crossed diplopia at near. His symptoms occur almost every day and are worse when he is tired. Your examination reveals an uncorrected acuity in each eye of 20/20. On a distant accommodative target, he is orthophoric. On a target at 1/3 m, he has a 15-prism-diopter exophoria. His near point of accommodation is 8 diopters in each eye. His fusional convergence amplitudes are 16 prism diopters to break and 12 to recover at 1/3 m, and 4 prism diopters to break and 2 to recover on a target at 6 m. Cycloplegic refraction reveals +0.75 sphere OD and +1.00 sphere OS.

The *best* treatment option is

a. correction of the cycloplegic refractive error
b. exercises for convergence insufficiency
c. glasses with base-in prisms
d. resection of both medial rectus muscles

P43 A 3-year-old girl has an esotropia that measures 18 prism diopters in primary position, 5 prism diopters in up gaze, and 35 prism diopters in down gaze. The ocular versions are shown in the figure. You plan to recess both medial rectus muscles for the esotropia.

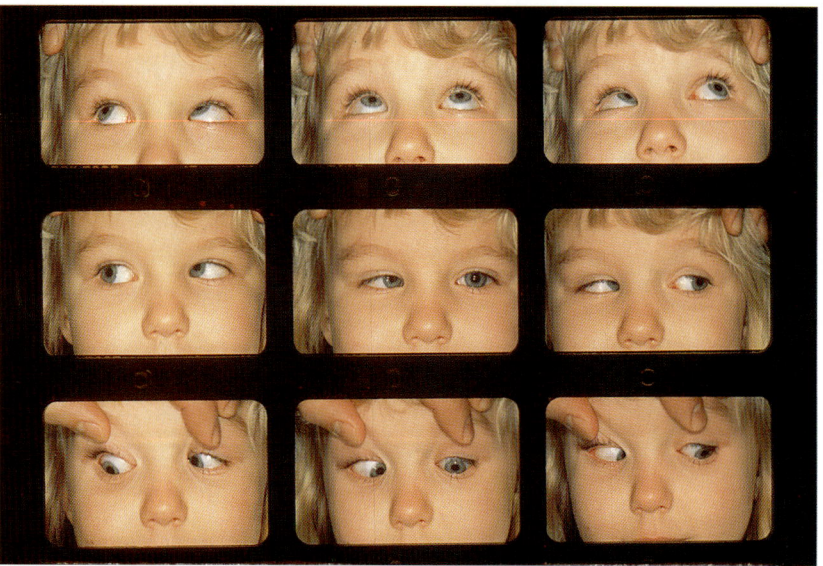

How would you manage the V pattern?

a. Weaken both inferior oblique muscles.
b. Infraplace both medial rectus muscles.
c. Reassess the V pattern after correcting the horizontal deviation in primary gaze.
d. Perform bilateral superior oblique tenotomies.

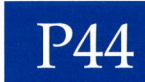

P44 A mother brings her 7-year-old son to you because he seems to be having trouble learning to spell and read. He is behind by at least one grade level in those areas. His math and art work are appropriate for his grade level. The patient's father had difficulty with school work as a child and currently wears glasses. The patient demonstrates 20/20 visual acuity in both eyes with a chart at 20 ft, but complains of difficulty with a near card and reads no better than 20/40. Your examination reveals +1.50 sphere OU and an exophoria of 2 prism diopters at near. Accommodative amplitudes and convergence fusional amplitudes are normal.

Which of the following statements is true?

a. The patient would benefit from orthoptic exercises.
b. The patient is probably going through a normal maturation process.
c. The patient should be evaluated for a possible learning disorder.
d. The patient should be treated with his hyperopic correction and a bifocal add.

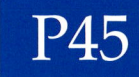

P45 Regarding developmental dyslexia, which of the following statements is true?

a. Dyslexia is not common in juvenile delinquents.
b. Dyslexics often present to ophthalmologists with visual symptoms.
c. Dyslexics rarely have a positive family history for dyslexia.
d. Dyslexics often have below-normal intelligence.

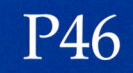

P46 A 7-year-old boy presents with a 9-month history of frequent episodes of blinking. The episodes are short in duration and occur randomly. Visual acuity is normal. The child's refractive error is +0.50 sphere in each eye. The remainder of the ocular examination is normal.

Which of the following statements is true?

a. A tear secretion test with and without anesthetic is likely to be diagnostic.
b. A conjunctival scraping to look for eosinophils and mast cells is indicated.
c. The blinking is most likely a habit.
d. The patient is likely to have a tic disorder.

P47 A 29-year-old woman has a history of esotropia that was diagnosed at 4 years of age and treated with glasses and patching for a few months. She has had decreased vision in her right eye for as long as she can remember. She has noticed more crossing of her right eye in the past few years and would like it corrected. Her best-corrected visual acuity is 20/100 OD with a –0.50 sphere and 20/20 OS with a +0.50 sphere. Your examination reveals a 20-prism-diopter right esotropia in primary and side gaze. The esotropia decreases to 5 prism diopters in up gaze and increases to 30 prism diopters in down gaze. The remainder of her ocular examination is normal.

Which of the following would be the *best* procedure to correct this deviation?

a. resection of the right lateral rectus muscle and recession of the right medial rectus muscle (R and R OD)
b. bilateral recessions of the medial rectus muscles with infraplacement
c. R and R OD with infraplacement of the medial rectus muscle and supraplacement of the lateral rectus muscle
d. R and R OD and a weakening procedure on the right inferior oblique muscle

P48 A 4½-year-old girl presents with a 3-week history of a red eye. The slit-lamp findings are shown in the figure. The eye has light-perception vision, and there is no view of the posterior pole. The other eye is normal.

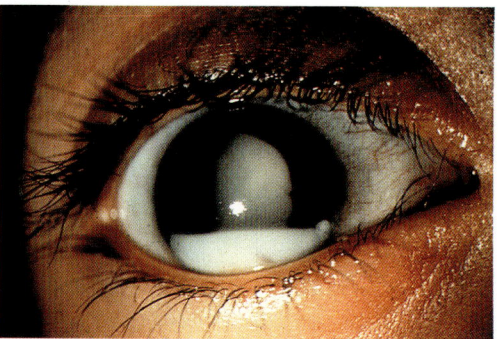

Appropriate investigation and management might include all of the following *except*

a. systemic evaluation for arthritis
b. angiotensin-converting enzyme (ACE) titer
c. an anterior chamber tap for cell identification and histopathology
d. CT scan of the head and orbits

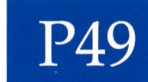 A 6-week-old infant presents to the ophthalmologist with a history of a bluish mass in the medial canthal area that has been present since birth (see the figure). A pediatric otorhinolaryngologist evaluated the patient and noted a mass lesion in the nose.

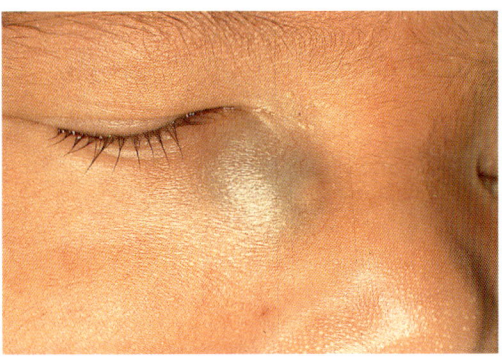

Which of the following is the *most* likely diagnosis?

a. nasal encephalocele
b. amniotocele
c. metastatic neuroblastoma
d. dermoid

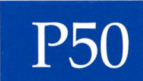 A 6-week-old infant was discharged from the hospital at 3 days of age with essentially the same appearance as shown in the figure. No further evaluation or treatment was recommended.

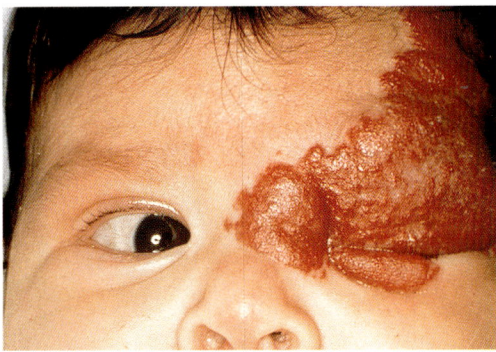

The *most* serious consequence of further lack of intervention in this child would be

a. metastatic disease and death
b. dense and irreversible amblyopia OS
c. permanent levator damage in the left upper eyelid
d. glaucoma OS

SECTION SEVEN
RETINA AND VITREOUS

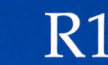 A healthy 28-year-old man presents with a 1-week history of pain, redness, and floaters in his left eye. Examination reveals visual acuity of 20/20 OD and 20/25 OS. The right eye is normal on examination. Significant findings on examination of the left eye are mild ciliary injection, fine keratic precipitates, mild anterior chamber cell, clear lens, and moderate anterior vitreous cell. The posterior pole appears normal except for a slightly hazy view secondary to vitreous debris. The lesion shown in the figure is present in the peripheral retina.

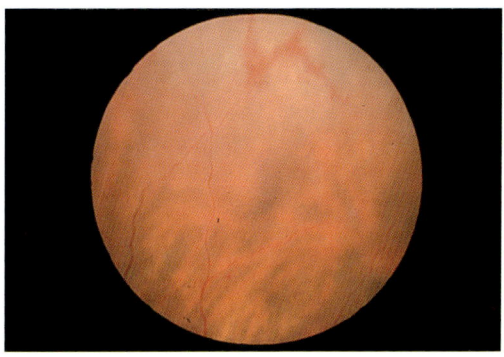

Given the patient's clinical presentation, what is the *most* likely diagnosis?

a. toxoplasmosis
b. cytomegalovirus retinitis
c. acute retinal necrosis syndrome
d. peripheral uveitis

 Following completion of the diagnostic workup, the *most* appropriate initial treatment for the patient in Question R1 is

a. intravenous acyclovir for a minimum of 5 to 10 days, followed by oral acyclovir
b. intravenous ganciclovir induction for 2 weeks, followed by daily maintenance ganciclovir
c. oral prednisone 60 mg to 80 mg per day
d. laser demarcation of peripheral retinal lesions

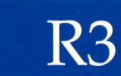 On routine ophthalmoscopic examination, a healthy 45-year-old woman is noted to have the retinal lesion depicted in the figure.

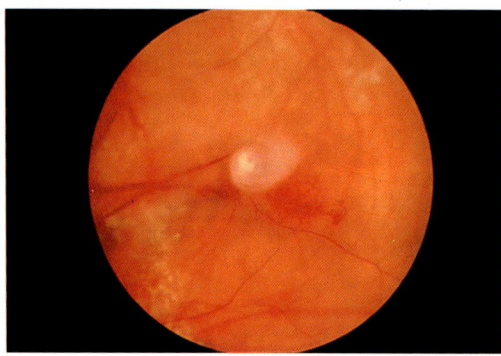

Which of the following courses of management is *most* appropriate?

a. Observe the lesion for change; no additional evaluation is necessary.
b. Ablate the lesion by laser photocoagulation or cryotherapy. If a detailed family history is negative, no additional evaluation is necessary.
c. Observe the lesion. Order a CT scan or MRI of the head, abdomen, and upper cervical spinal cord and obtain a detailed family history.
d. Ablate the lesion by laser photocoagulation or cryotherapy. Regardless of the findings of a detailed family history, order a CT scan or MRI of the head, abdomen, and upper cervical spinal cord.

 All of the following are risk factors for the development of neovascular age-related macular degeneration *except*

a. increased serum cholesterol level
b. cigarette smoking
c. exogenous estrogen use in postmenopausal women
d. soft drusen

 A 72-year-old woman presents with metamorphopsia and blurred vision OD of 1 month's duration. On examination, her visual acuity is 20/30 OD and 20/20 OS. Mild cataract is present symmetrically in both eyes. In the posterior pole OD, a large, smooth, dome-shaped elevation is noted without associated hemorrhage, lipid, or serous retinal detachment. Soft drusen are scattered in the posterior pole of both eyes. The early view (see the figure, part A) and late view (see the figure, part B) of the fluorescein angiogram are shown.

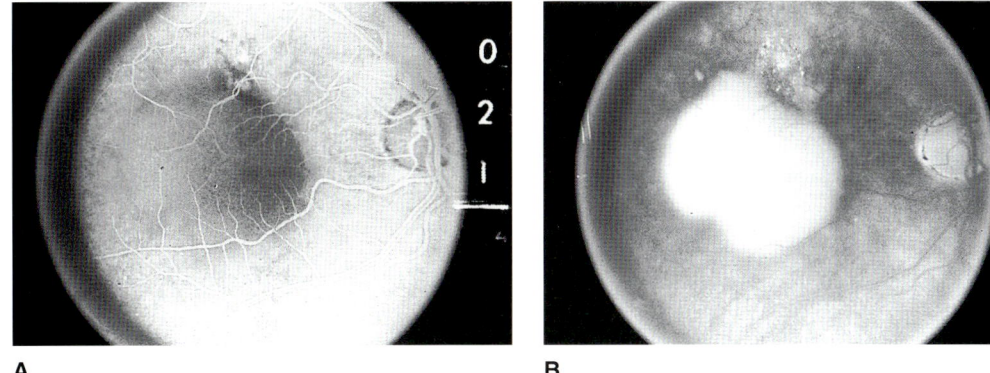

A B

All of the following statements regarding the patient's condition are correct *except*

a. Indocyanine green angiography may be helpful in further assessing this patient.
b. This patient's risk of developing exudative age-related macular degeneration in her fellow eye is between 4% and 12% annually.
c. A retinal pigment epithelial tear may complicate treatment of this lesion.
d. There is angiographic evidence of choroidal neovascularization beneath the fovea.

R6 A 78-year-old man presents with the fundus and angiographic findings shown in the figures.

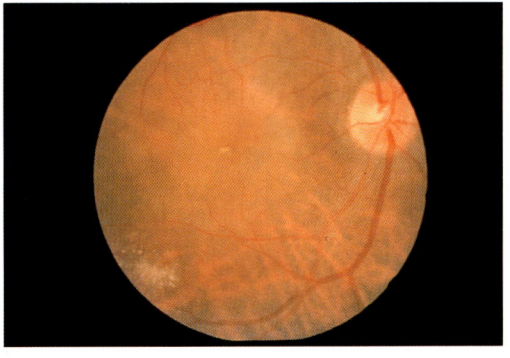
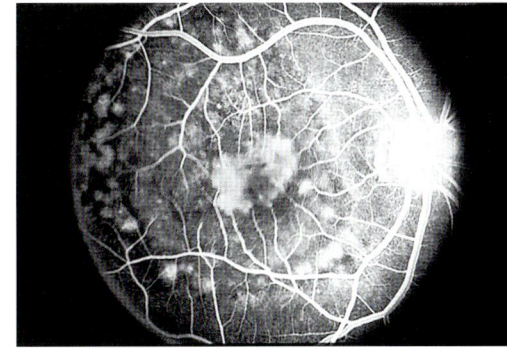

A B

Which of the following is *most* important in determining if treatment with laser photocoagulation should be recommended?

a. lesion size and initial visual acuity
b. a lesion with well-defined borders
c. a lesion with features of classic choroidal neovascularization
d. a disciform scar in the fellow eye

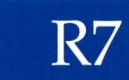 In the emergency room you are asked to examine the fundi of an obtunded 2-year-old girl who has no visible signs of external injury. She has no known prior medical problems. Examination reveals large, dome-shaped hemorrhages beneath the internal limiting membrane (ILM) in the posterior pole in both eyes (left eye shown in the figure). A few scattered retinal hemorrhages are visible in the retinal periphery of both eyes. A small, circumferential retinal fold extends around the margin of the sub-ILM hemorrhage in each eye.

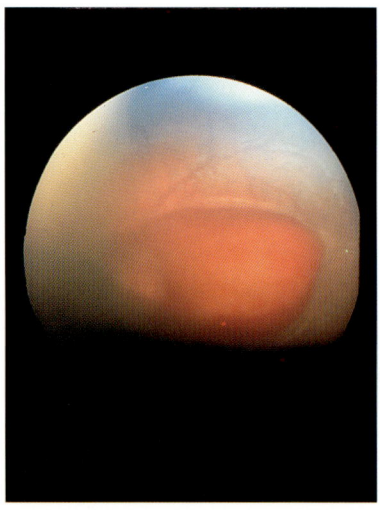

Which of the following is the *most* likely cause of the retinal abnormalities?

a. juvenile retinoschisis
b. acute myelogenous leukemia
c. child abuse
d. retinal macroaneurysm

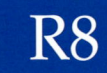 A 70-year-old woman presents for followup examination 2 months after trabeculectomy in her left eye. She is without complaints; her best-corrected visual acuity is 20/25 OU with −1.00 + 0.50 × 120 OD and −0.50 + 0.25 × 30 OS; IOP is 19 mm Hg OD and 13 mm Hg OS. External and ocular motility examinations are normal. A good filtering bleb is visible superonasally OS; the conjunctiva is white OU; the anterior chamber is quiet and deep OU; and mild nuclear sclerosis and cortical lens opacities are present OU. Fundus examination in the right eye is normal. The left fundus and corresponding fluorescein angiogram are shown in the figures.

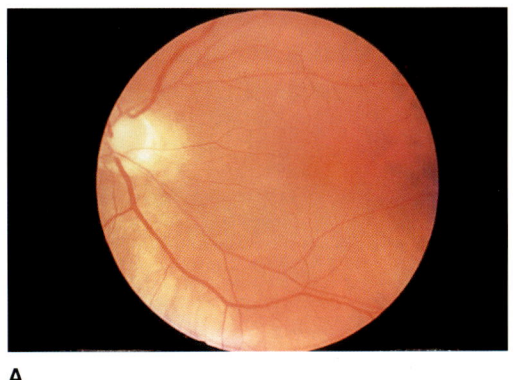
A

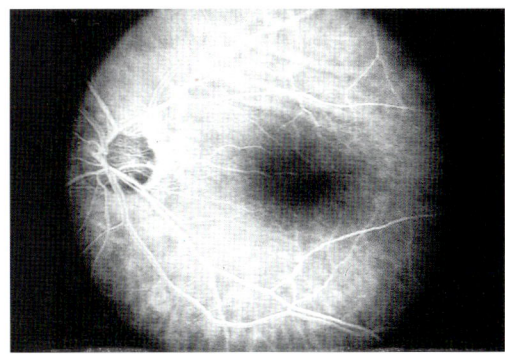
B

The choroidal abnormality is *most* likely the result of

a. choroidal neovascularization
b. retrobulbar tumor
c. previous hypotony
d. epiretinal membrane

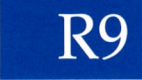 A 28-year-old man with acquired immunodeficiency syndrome (AIDS) presents with the right fundus shown in the figure.

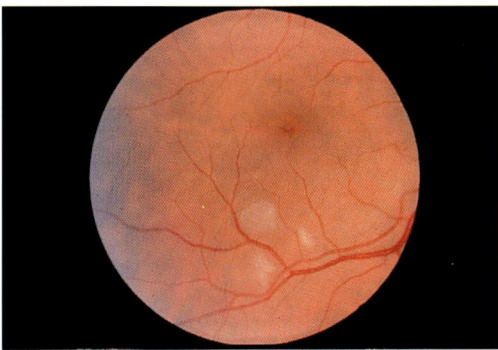

Which of the following statements regarding the patient's condition is *most* accurate?

a. The lesions most likely represent early CMV retinitis, if the patient's CD4 lymphocyte count is less than 50 cells/mm^3.
b. The lesions most likely are cotton-wool spots, which are a manifestation of human immunodeficiency virus (HIV)-related noninfectious retinal vasculopathy and do not require close followup.
c. The lesions may represent either cotton-wool spots or early CMV retinitis. Close observation of the patient for change in these lesions, with documentation of the fundus by photographs, is indicated.
d. If the patient is without symptoms and no retinal hemorrhage is associated with these lesions, they do not represent CMV retinitis.

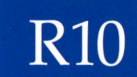 A 32-year-old man with a history of AIDS and CMV retinitis OU initially received ganciclovir but was switched to foscarnet 6 months later when recurrence of the CMV retinitis indicated resistance to ganciclovir. Following foscarnet therapy, all CMV activity in the retina resolved. The patient now presents with the fundus appearance shown in the figure. His creatinine clearance is currently reduced and his white blood cell count is critically low.

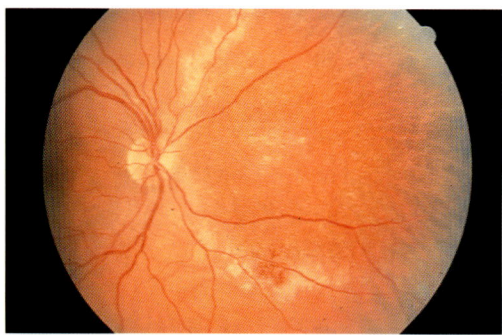

Which treatment plan would be the *most* desirable in this patient?

a. Stop intravenous foscarnet and either give intravitreal ganciclovir or foscarnet by injection, or use a sustained-release ganciclovir device intravitreally.
b. Repeat induction doses of foscarnet intravenously.
c. Continue foscarnet and start induction doses of ganciclovir intravenously.
d. Add zidovudine (AZT) to the current foscarnet therapy.

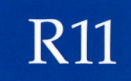 All of the following statements about central retinal artery occlusion are true *except*

a. Electroretinography shows a diminished A-wave.
b. Long-term survival is decreased in patients who have had retinal artery occlusions.
c. Iris neovascularization may occur in 5% of patients.
d. Emboli more commonly cause retinal arterial occlusions than thrombosis or vascular narrowing from atherosclerosis.

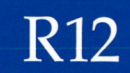 An 84-year-old woman with a history of bilateral pseudophakia presents with a 7-day history of sudden, decreased vision in her right eye without associated pain, redness, or photophobia. Examination reveals best-corrected visual acuity of counting fingers at 2 feet OD and 20/25 OS. Examination of the right eye shows an afferent pupillary defect, inferior keratic precipitates, and mild flare and cell. The vitreous in the right eye contains clumps of white, cellular debris. The right fundus is shown in the figure. Posterior chamber IOLs are in position with central posterior capsular openings OU. The left eye is normal. The patient was diagnosed 4 years ago with tuberculosis and was treated medically for it for 1 year.

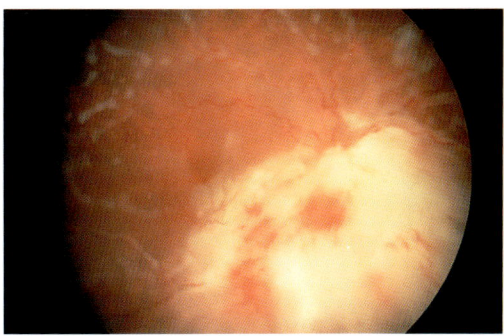

Which of the following is *least* likely to be helpful in establishing a diagnosis in this patient?

a. fluorescein angiography
b. vitreous biopsy for cytology and microbiology
c. magnetic resonance imaging (MRI) of the head and orbits
d. referral to an internist for evaluation of possible systemic malignancy, immunosuppression, or reactivation of tuberculosis

R13 A vitreous biopsy of the patient in Question R12 demonstrates cryptococcal organisms on fungal stain and culture. All of the following statements about endogenous ocular cryptococcal infections are true *except*

a. Cryptococcal meningitis is frequently associated with ocular cryptococcal infections.
b. Cryptococcal infections occur only in immunosuppressed patients.
c. Ocular involvement frequently is the result of direct extension along the optic nerve or by hematogenous spread.
d. Chorioretinitis is the most common intraocular presentation of *Cryptococcus*.

R14 A 24-year-old man with a 10-year history of insulin-dependent diabetes mellitus presents with a visual acuity of 20/25 OD and 20/200 OS. Examination of the macula in the right eye demonstrates hard exudate and retinal thickening to within 500 microns of the foveal center. A small area of flat retinal neovascularization is present in the right eye off the superotemporal arcade. The vitreous in the right eye is clear. Examination of the left eye demonstrates diffuse retinal thickening throughout the macula, scattered hard exudates, and blot hemorrhages. Marked neovascularization of the disc is present in the left eye, as well as nasal retinal neovascularization with mild vitreous hemorrhage.

The *best* sequence of photocoagulation treatment for this patient is

a. initial focal photocoagulation OU, followed by panretinal photocoagulation OU
b. initial panretinal photocoagulation OU, followed by focal photocoagulation OS
c. initial panretinal photocoagulation OS, followed by focal photocoagulation OU
d. initial panretinal and focal photocoagulation OS, followed by focal photocoagulation OD

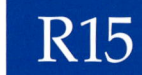

The Diabetes Control and Complications Trial was a multicenter, randomized clinical trial in which insulin-dependent diabetic patients with either no retinopathy or mild to moderate nonproliferative retinopathy were treated either with conventional insulin therapy or intensive insulin therapy that consisted of either three or more insulin injections daily or an insulin pump.

All of the following statements about the findings of this trial are true *except*

a. In patients initially without retinopathy, intensive insulin therapy reduced the risk of onset of retinopathy by 76% compared to patients in the conventional therapy group.
b. In patients initially with mild to moderate nonproliferative retinopathy, intensive insulin therapy slowed the progression of retinopathy by 54% compared to patients in the conventional therapy group.
c. In patients with mild to moderate nonproliferative retinopathy, intensive therapy reduced the development of proliferative or severe nonproliferative retinopathy by 47% compared to conventional insulin therapy.
d. No transient early worsening of retinopathy with intensive insulin therapy was noted in patients with mild to moderate retinopathy, as reported in previous trials.

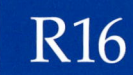

A 60-year-old hypertensive woman with insulin-dependent diabetes mellitus of 27 years' duration presents with complaints of gradual decrease in visual acuity in her right eye. On examination, her visual acuity is 20/60 OD and 20/30 OS. Previously, she had laser photocoagulation for clinically significant diabetic macular edema OU. The fundus photograph (see the figure, part A) and fluorescein angiogram (see the figure, part B) for the right eye are shown.

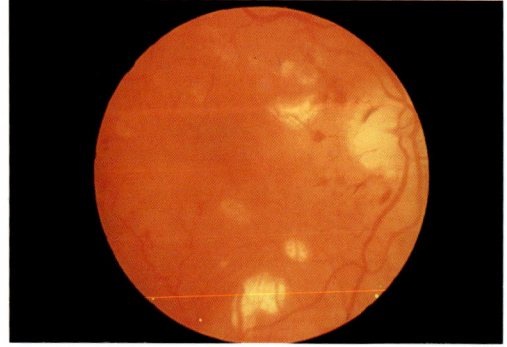
A

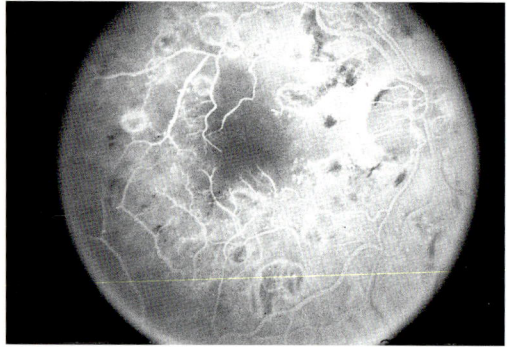
B

Which of the following statements about this patient is *most* accurate?

a. Focal laser photocoagulation OD is the treatment of choice.
b. There is no visible abnormality on either the fundus photograph or fluorescein angiogram OD to explain the patient's decrease in visual acuity. Therefore, optic nerve dysfunction should be considered.
c. Macular ischemia most likely accounts for the patient's decrease in visual acuity in the right eye.
d. Modified grid photocoagulation OD is the treatment of choice.

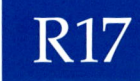

All of the following statements about *Propionibacterium acnes* endophthalmitis are correct *except*

a. *Propionibacterium* may cause a recurrent granulomatous iridocyclitis that may not develop until months after cataract surgery.
b. Nd:YAG laser capsulotomy may cause a flare-up of the intraocular inflammation in *Propionibacterium* endophthalmitis.
c. *Propionibacterium acnes* is frequently found in the normal flora of the conjunctiva.
d. Inflammation associated with *Propionibacterium* endophthalmitis typically increases with topical corticosteroid use.

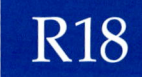

A 74-year-old woman who underwent trabeculectomy in her left eye 2 years ago for primary open-angle glaucoma presents with a 2-day history of decreased vision and redness OS. On examination, her visual acuity is 20/25 OD and 20/200 OS. Intraocular pressure is 15 mm Hg OD and 22 mm Hg OS. The slit-lamp appearance OS is shown in the figure. A 1 mm hypopyon and moderate vitreous cell are also present.

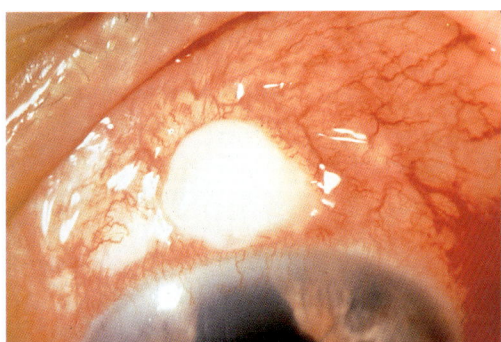

Which of the following statements regarding the patient's condition is *least* correct?

a. It is unusual to see this complication after filtration surgery unless the filtration bleb is Seidel-positive.
b. *Streptococcus* or *Haemophilus* organisms are most commonly associated with this condition.
c. Closed vitrectomy with injection of broad-spectrum intravitreal antibiotics such as an aminoglycoside and vancomycin would be an appropriate course of management in this patient.
d. Filtering procedures using antimetabolites such as 5-fluorouracil have a higher risk of this complication.

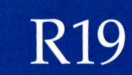 In the evaluation and treatment of diabetic retinopathy, fluorescein angiography is *least* useful

a. to determine areas of capillary closure
b. to determine the presence of clinically significant diabetic macular edema prior to recommending photocoagulation
c. to determine the location of diffuse retinal leakage from incompetent retinal capillaries or intraretinal microvascular abnormalities prior to photocoagulation
d. to determine the location of retinal microaneurysms prior to photocoagulation

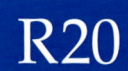 A 26-year-old myopic man presents with a 5-day history of photopsias, small scotomas, and blurred vision in both eyes. He is recovering from a recent flu-like illness. Examination reveals best-corrected visual acuity of 20/50 OD and 20/40 OS. Slit-lamp examination shows mild flare and cell in both anterior chambers and mild vitreous cell in both eyes. The fundus findings are similar in both eyes; the right fundus is shown in the figure.

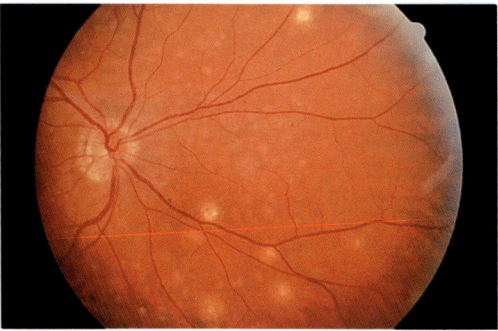

Which of the following diagnoses is *most* likely in this patient?

a. presumed ocular histoplasmosis syndrome
b. multifocal choroiditis
c. birdshot retinochoroidopathy
d. acute posterior multifocal placoid pigment epitheliopathy

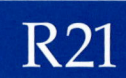 A 32-year-old man presents without complaints for routine examination. On indirect ophthalmoscopy, multiple patches of peripheral lattice degeneration containing multiple atrophic retinal holes are noted in the superior retina OD. Lattice degeneration without retinal breaks is noted inferiorly OS. Which of the following statements regarding prophylactic treatment is *most* correct?

a. Only the patient's right eye should be prophylactically treated with laser photocoagulation or cryoretinopexy.
b. Both of the patient's eyes should be prophylactically treated with laser photocoagulation or cryoretinopexy.
c. If there is a prior history of retinal detachment in the left eye, prophylactic laser photocoagulation or cryoretinopexy should be considered in the right eye.
d. The patient's right eye should receive prophylactic treatment with laser photocoagulation or cryoretinopexy prior to cataract surgery.

R22 A 12-year-old boy presents with a nonpenetrating BB gun injury in the right eye. His visual acuity is 20/400 OD and 20/20 OS. Slit-lamp examination reveals a focal conjunctival hemorrhage temporally OD with no evidence of scleral laceration. The anterior segment appears normal except for moderate cell and flare OD. Mild diffuse vitreous hemorrhage is present with dense hemorrhage inferiorly OD. Retinal examination OD reveals an area of hemorrhagic and necrotic retina temporally with accompanying RPE and choroidal disruption and bare sclera visible, as shown in the figure. Commotio retinae surrounds the area of retinal and choroidal loss and extends into the macula. Cystoid edema is present in the macula. No other retinal breaks are visible, although vitreous hemorrhage prevents complete examination of the peripheral retina.

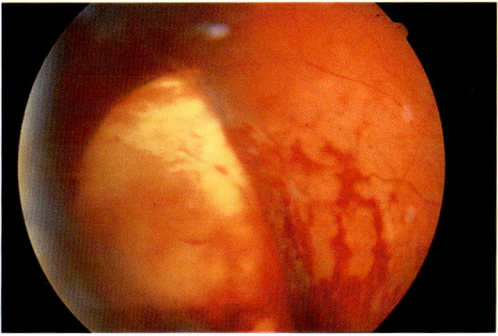

Which of the following is *least* likely to result in later decreased visual acuity in this patient?

a. retinal detachment resulting from the necrotic retinal break
b. retinal detachment resulting from a peripheral retinal break, if present
c. granular pigmentation in the macula following resolution of the commotio retinae
d. macular hole

R23 Indications for immediate or early pars plana vitrectomy in a penetrating injury include all of the following *except*

a. intraocular foreign body
b. early endophthalmitis
c. retinal detachment with vitreous hemorrhage
d. vitreous incarceration in a posterior scleral wound that cannot be closed by an external approach

R24 All of the following statements about peripheral uveitis are true *except*

a. The most common causes of reduction in visual acuity in peripheral uveitis are cystoid macular edema and vitreous debris.
b. Fluorescein angiography may demonstrate staining of peripheral retinal vessels.
c. An indication for initiating treatment for peripheral uveitis is a reduction in visual acuity to less than 20/25.
d. Lyme disease, Fuchs' heterochromic cyclitis, *Toxocara canis*, toxoplasmosis, and retinoblastoma are included in the differential diagnosis of peripheral uveitis.

R25 A healthy 22-year-old man presents with a 6-month history of floaters OU and a 1-month history of painless decrease in visual acuity OS. Examination reveals a visual acuity of 20/25 OD and 20/50 OS, no injection, quiet anterior chamber, clear lens, mild to moderate anterior vitreous cell, and a thick white deposit of debris over the inferior ora serrata/pars plana in both eyes. The figures show the patient's fundus appearance (part A) and fluorescein angiogram (part B) of the left eye. Systemic evaluation, including chest x-ray, PPD, FTA-ABS, and titers for *Toxoplasma*, Lyme disease, and *Toxocara canis*, is normal.

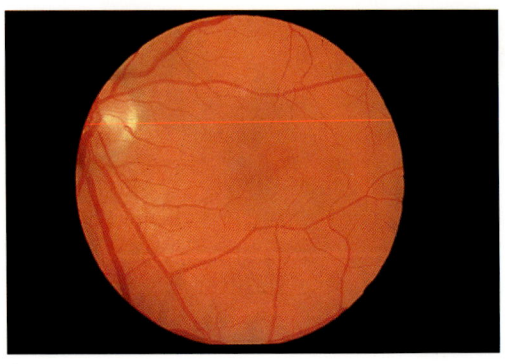
A

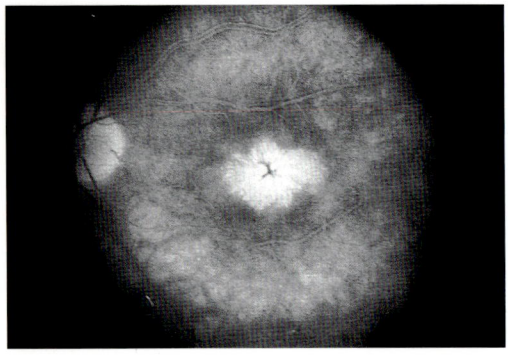
B

Initial treatment should consist of

a. systemic prednisone beginning at 60 mg po qd for 2 weeks
b. topical prednisolone acetate OS
c. posterior subtenon's or transseptal injection of corticosteroid OS
d. cryotherapy to the area of pars plana debris OS

R26 All of the following statements about retinal detachment patient selection for pneumatic retinopexy are true *except*

a. Retinal break(s) should be located within the superior two-thirds of the fundus.
b. Retinal break(s) should be located within 1 clock hour of each other.
c. Patients with proliferative vitreoretinopathy (PVR) grade C or higher or severe glaucoma should not be considered candidates for pneumatic retinopexy.
d. Aphakic or pseudophakic patients have the same rate of success with pneumatic retinopexy as phakic patients.

R27 A 60-year-old man presents with a 3-day history of photopsias and new floaters in his left eye. His visual acuity is 20/20 OU. Slit-lamp examination shows mild nuclear sclerosis and clear anterior vitreous bilaterally. On fundus examination, a posterior vitreous detachment (PVD) is seen only in the left eye.

All of the following statements are true *except*

a. If hemorrhage or pigment granules are not present in the vitreous, depressed examination of the peripheral retina is not necessary.
b. Approximately 15% of patients who present with acute, symptomatic PVD will have a retinal tear.
c. In the majority of cases, when the fellow eye develops a PVD it will likely respond in the same way (ie, symptoms, complications) as the first eye did upon developing PVD.
d. Myopia, diabetic retinopathy, vitreous hemorrhage, and surgical aphakia all predispose the patient to vitreous detachment at an earlier age.

R28 An increased rate of proliferative vitreoretinopathy (PVR) has been associated with all of the following *except*

a. vitreous hemorrhage
b. scleral buckling surgery rather than closed vitrectomy for the repair of retinal detachment
c. large and/or multiple retinal breaks
d. cryoretinopexy

R29 All of the following statements about the use of indirect ophthalmoscopy to screen for retinopathy of prematurity are true *except*

a. Screening should be performed prior to hospital discharge or by 4 to 6 weeks of age.
b. Screening should be performed on all premature neonates of less than 30 weeks' gestation.
c. Screening should be performed on all premature neonates with a birth weight of less than 1300 g.
d. Screening should be repeated biweekly on neonates who demonstrate retinopathy of prematurity on the initial examination.

R30 On routine ophthalmoscopic examination, a 62-year-old woman is noted to have asymptomatic, bilateral, smooth peripheral elevations in the inferotemporal retina that extend slightly posterior to the equator. Visual acuity is 20/20 OU. Which of the following statements is true?

a. Laser demarcation along the posterior border of these lesions will prevent extension into the macula.
b. Retinal detachment frequently occurs in such a case if an inner-layer retinal break is present.
c. Retinal detachment will not occur unless a retinal break is present in the outer layer or full-thickness retina.
d. Retinal detachments associated with outer-layer breaks typically progress rapidly.

R31 The results of an ultrasound test are shown in the figure.

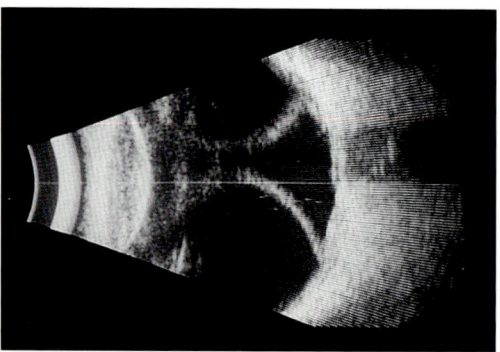

All of the following statements about this nonmobile ultrasound finding are true *except*

a. Surgical drainage is indicated in most cases.
b. Excessive panretinal photocoagulation may produce this lesion.
c. A shallow anterior chamber may be associated with this lesion.
d. A double-peaked spike is a characteristic finding observed on A-scan.

R32 A 54-year-old woman complains that 1 month ago she developed metamorphopsia, followed by a sudden decrease in central vision in her left eye. Her visual acuity is 20/20 OD and 20/100 OS. Anterior segment examination demonstrates trace nuclear sclerosis OU. Her fundi are shown in the figures.

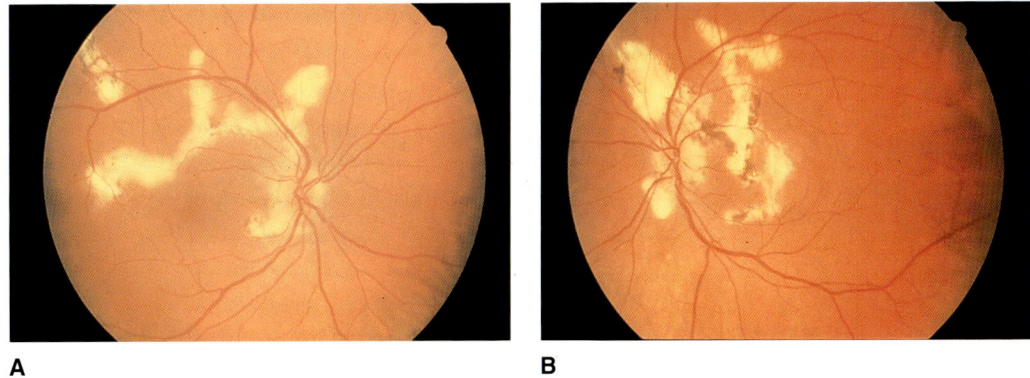

All of the following statements about this patient's ocular condition are true *except*

a. Visual loss may occur from progression of this condition into the fovea.
b. Visual loss may occur from a secondary subretinal neovascular membrane involving the fovea.
c. Visual loss may occur secondary to optic nerve involvement.
d. Recurrences are common and typically progress outward from the optic disc from the edge of old lesions.

R33

A 67-year-old woman presents with a history of uncomplicated extracapsular cataract extraction with a posterior chamber IOL in her left eye 3 years ago and bilateral iritis beginning 2 years ago. Visual acuity is 20/40 OD and 20/25 OS. Slit-lamp examination shows quiet anterior chambers OU, mild nuclear sclerosis OD, and a posterior chamber IOL in good position with a central posterior capsular opening OS. Mild anterior vitreous cell is present OU. The patient's fundi are shown in the figures. Fluorescein angiography confirms cystoid macular edema OU and scattered postequatorial hypofluorescent lesions corresponding to the hypopigmented lesions in the fundus photographs.

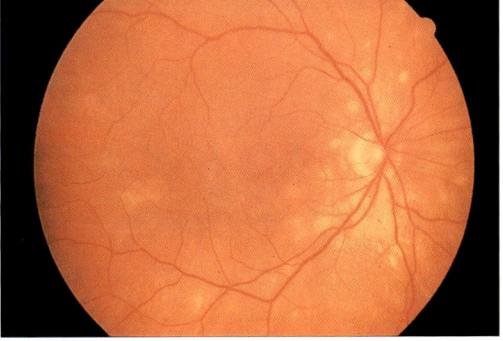
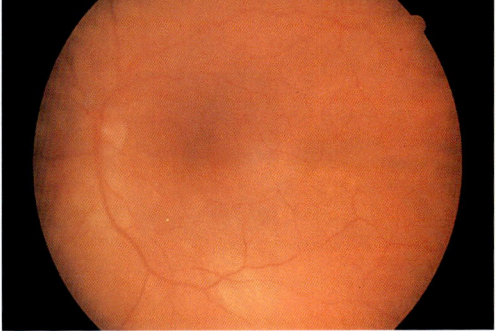

All of the following statements about this patient's condition are true *except*

a. HLA-A29 antigen is frequently present.
b. Serous retinal detachments may be seen.
c. Most such patients respond poorly to corticosteroid therapy.
d. Although visual acuity may be affected, most such patients retain useful central vision in at least one eye for many years.

R34 A 67-year-old woman presents with a 1-week history of sudden, painless loss of vision in her right eye. She notes no preceding or associated symptoms. She has hypertension that is controlled by medication but no history of diabetes mellitus. On examination, her visual acuity is counting fingers at 1 foot OD and 20/20 OS. Anterior segment examination is normal. Fundus examination reveals a dense vitreous hemorrhage OD. The left fundus exam demonstrates a few drusen in the macula but no other abnormalities. Ultrasonography of the right eye is shown in the figure.

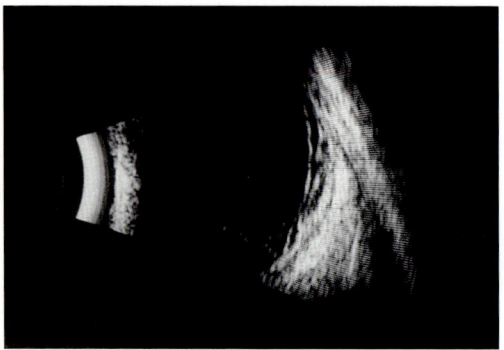

The *least* likely cause for her vitreous hemorrhage is

a. retinal tear
b. retinal vein occlusion
c. melanoma
d. extramacular disciform lesion

R35 A subfoveal yellow lesion in the macula of a 62-year-old woman is shown in the fundus photograph (see the figure, part A) and fluorescein angiogram (see the figure, part B).

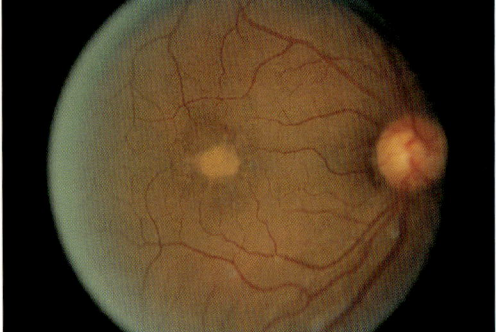 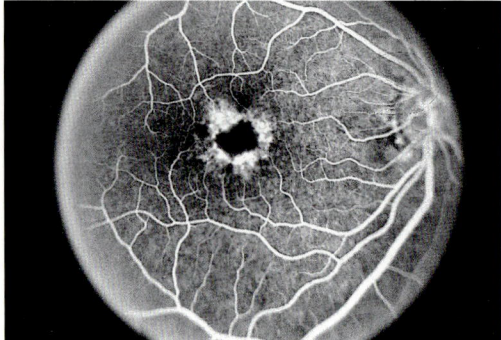

A B

Which of the following is true?

a. The lesion is typically associated with severely decreased visual acuity.
b. The lesion has a high risk of developing choroidal neovascularization.
c. The lesion is typically hypofluorescent on fluorescein angiography and is surrounded by an incomplete ring of hyperfluorescence that fades in the late angiogram.
d. The lesion is likely to undergo rapid changes with time.

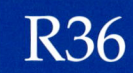

Following an uneventful cataract extraction, a 66-year-old woman is referred to you because of an elevated gray choroidal mass in her left eye. Her left eye has a visual acuity of 20/25 and shows no evidence of inflammation. In the superior periphery, there is a large, dome-shaped, gray choroidal mass as shown in the figure, part A. A minimal amount of subretinal fluid is present around the margins of the lesion. Echographic examination (see the figure, parts B and C) shows that the lesion has a regular internal acoustic pattern and is of very low reflectivity.

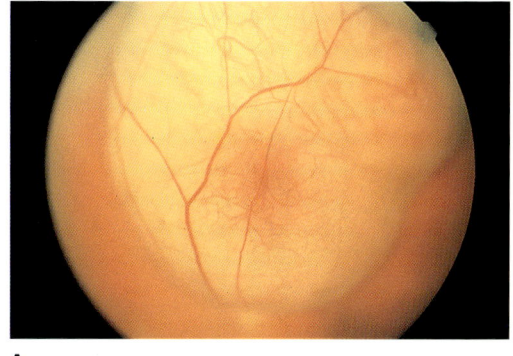

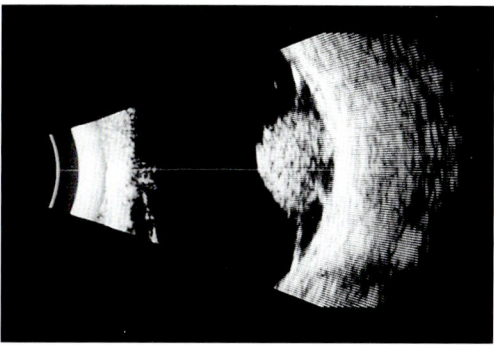

The choroidal mass is *most* consistent with

a. scleritis
b. choroidal detachment
c. choroidal metastasis
d. amelanotic choroidal melanoma

R37 A 64-year-old man is referred to you because of an elevated, brown choroidal mass involving the inferior quadrant of his left eye. On echographic examination, the lesion shows a pattern highly consistent with malignant melanoma. A subsequent metastatic workup is completely negative.

Factors predictive of subsequent metastatic disease include all of the following *except*

a. cell type
b. extrascleral extension
c. extension through Bruch's membrane
d. location of the anterior tumor margin

R38 A 60-year-old man has bilateral graying of the retina temporal to the fovea (see the figure, part A), subtle angiographic evidence of staining in this area (see the figure, part B), and visual acuity of 20/25 OU.

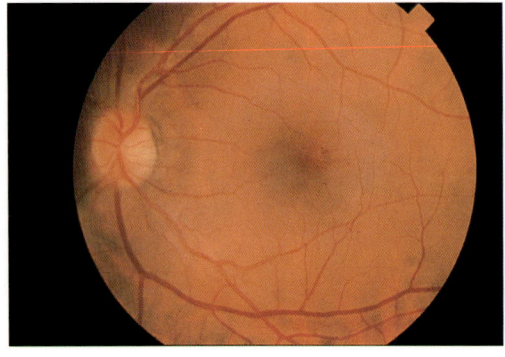 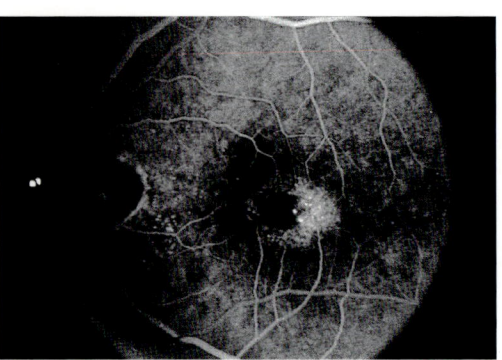

A				B

The *most* likely diagnosis is

a. cone dystrophy
b. age-related macular degeneration
c. idiopathic juxtafoveolar retinal telangiectasis
d. chloroquine toxicity

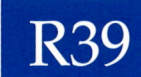

R39 The *early* manifestations of the condition diagnosed in Question R38 include all of the following *except*

a. pigmentary migration into the retina
b. temporal graying of the macula
c. a diffuse pattern of late staining surrounding the fovea on fluorescein angiography
d. asymmetric presentation

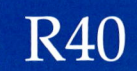

R40 A patient with diabetes presents with an optic disc appearance as shown in the figure.

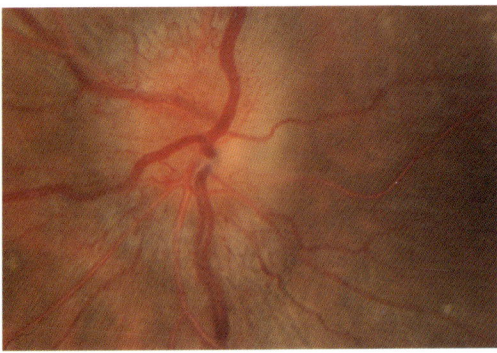

Which of the following statements about the condition illustrated is true?

a. It only afflicts patients in diabetic ketoacidosis.
b. It usually causes severe and permanent visual acuity loss.
c. It is characterized by disc edema in one or both eyes.
d. It is treated with panretinal photocoagulation.

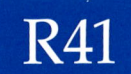

R41 The parents of a 2-year-old girl report that she has had "bobbing eyes" and light sensitivity since birth. In your office, the girl shows good visual attention but has bilateral pendular nystagmus and squints in bright light. The retina appears normal, but the foveal reflex is blunted. Dark-adapted scotopic electroretinogram (ERG) responses are normal, but light-adapted photopic signals are greatly diminished. No relatives are similarly affected.

This patient *most* likely has

a. congenital stationary night blindness (CSNB)
b. Leber's congenital amaurosis
c. achromatopsia
d. Stargardt's disease

R42 A 12-year-old boy fails his school vision screening test. His medical history is benign. Middle-aged relatives of both sexes for three generations reportedly have had central visual loss. His best-corrected visual acuities are 20/80 OD and 20/20 OS. The disc, vessels, and retinal periphery of both eyes appear normal but the macula of the right eye has a fibrotic scar and the left eye shows a yellow, round, circumscribed lesion of one disc diameter (see the figure) that blocks fluorescence on fluorescein angiogram. The ERG is normal, but the electrooculogram ratio (light peak/dark trough) is reduced.

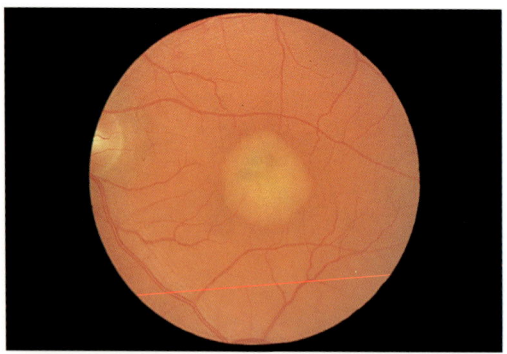

The *most* likely diagnosis is

a. neuronal ceroid lipofuscinosis
b. Bardet-Biedl syndrome
c. Best's vitelliform macular dystrophy
d. Stargardt's disease

R43 A 47-year-old woman in good health with a history of autosomal dominant retinitis pigmentosa presents with complaints of further decline in visual acuity in both eyes. On examination, her visual acuity is 20/100 OD and 20/70 OS. Mild posterior subcapsular cataract is present in both lenses. Moderate fine cell is seen on biomicroscopy of the vitreous of both eyes. The fundi are shown in the figures (right eye: parts A and B; left eye: parts C and D). The patient's sister has retinitis pigmentosa that required retinal laser treatment 2 years earlier.

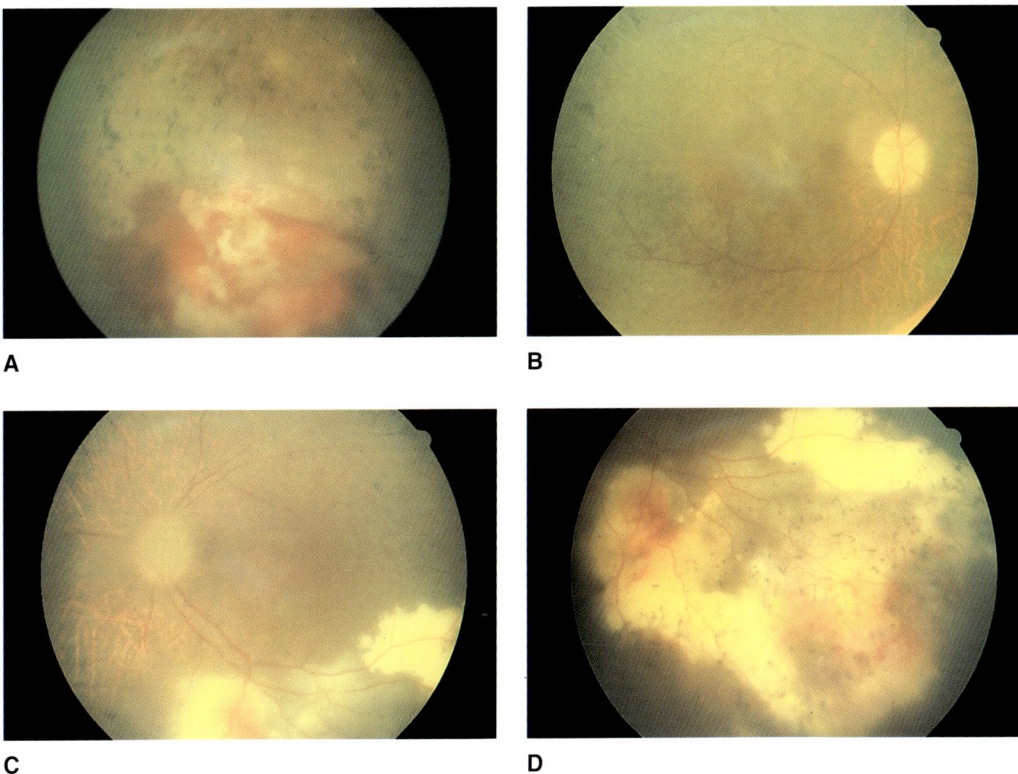

Which of the following statements regarding this patient is *most* correct?

a. The patient's clinical appearance is most characteristic of Coats' retinopathy, which may occur in retinitis pigmentosa.
b. The subretinal exudates most likely are the result of retinal infection with toxoplasmosis.
c. The patient's clinical appearance is most characteristic of familial exudative vitreoretinopathy.
d. The retinal findings most likely result from diabetes mellitus, and a glucose tolerance test should be performed.

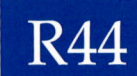 A 60-year-old hypertensive woman presents with sudden loss of vision in her right eye. Her visual acuity is counting fingers OD and 20/30 OS. Ophthalmoscopy of the left eye reveals arteriolar narrowing and severe arteriovenous crossing nicks. No drusen are seen OS. The right fundus (part A) and fluorescein angiogram (part B) are shown in the figures.

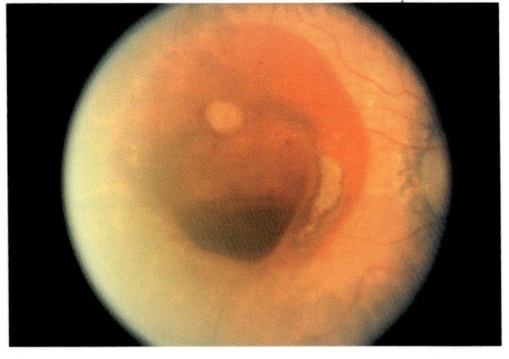
A

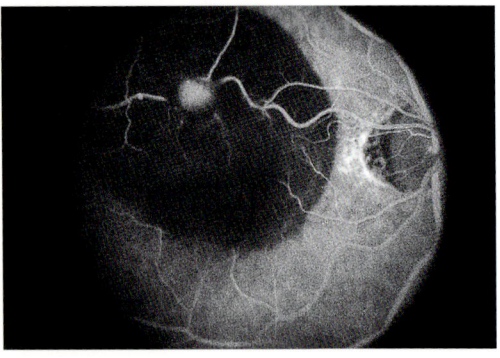
B

The *most* likely diagnosis is

a. age-related macular degeneration
b. retinal artery macroaneurysm
c. idiopathic choroidal neovascular membrane
d. choroidal rupture

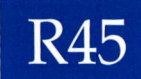 A 65-year-old woman presents for evaluation of recent visual loss in her right eye. Her visual acuity is 20/40 OD and 20/20 OS. Biomicroscopy of the macula is shown in the figure.

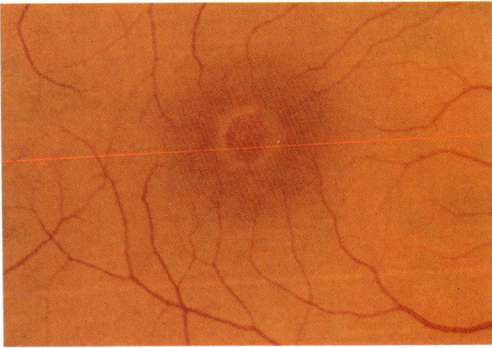

All of the following are true *except*

a. Amsler grid examination is likely to show metamorphopsia.
b. Posterior vitreous detachment is unlikely to be present in the right eye.
c. There is a 40% to 50% chance that the lesion will resolve spontaneously.
d. The patient has a greater than 50% chance of developing a similar problem in the fellow eye.

Section Seven: Retina and Vitreous

R46 A 70-year-old woman complains of progressive blurring in her right eye. Examination is unremarkable apart from mild vitreous cell and the nodular, shallowly elevated lesion shown in the figures (part A, temporal retina; part B, posterior pole).

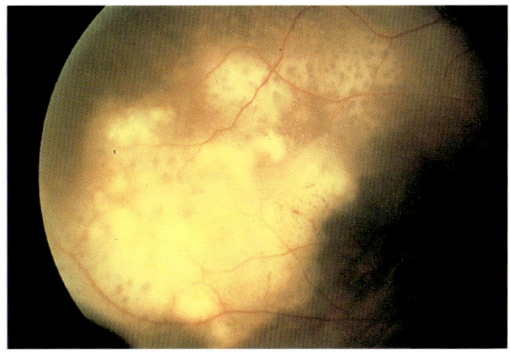

A

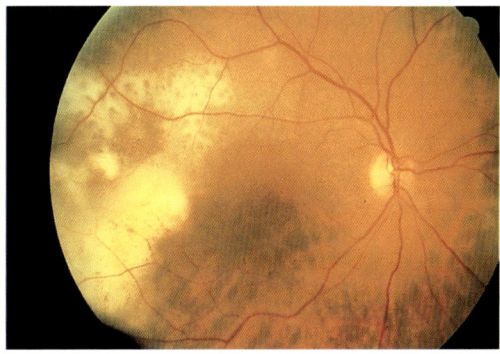

B

The *most* likely diagnosis is

a. amelanotic melanoma of the choroid
b. tuberculous choroiditis
c. intraocular lymphoma
d. carcinoma metastatic to the choroid

R47 A 10-year-old girl is brought to see you with complaints of decreased vision and headache over the preceding 4 to 6 weeks. Fundus findings are shown in the figures.

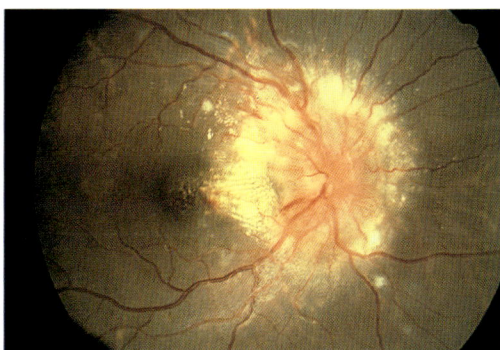

A

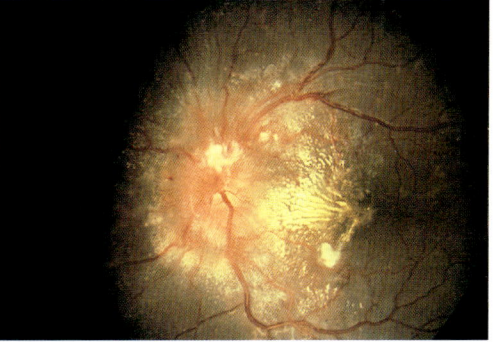

B

C

Which of the following tests should be performed *first*?

a. CT scan of the head
b. systemic blood pressure measurement
c. lumbar puncture
d. FTA-ABS test

R48 An otherwise healthy, emmetropic 45-year-old man reports gradually diminishing vision in his right eye. There is no history of surgery, trauma, or laser treatment. Ocular examination demonstrates dilated episcleral veins, normal intraocular pressure, mild vitreous cells, shallow peripheral ciliochoroidal detachment, nonrhegmatogenous retinal detachment with markedly shifting subretinal fluid, and the pigment alterations shown in the fundus photograph (see the figure, part A) and fluorescein angiogram (see the figure, part B). There are no intraocular masses or signs of significant ocular inflammation.

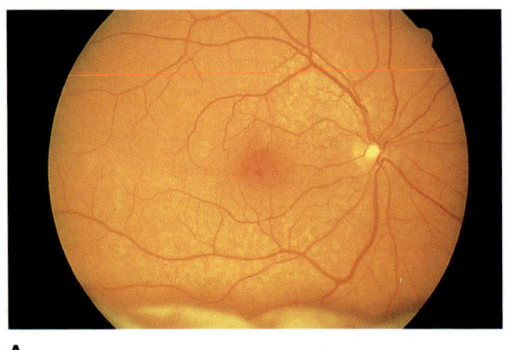
A

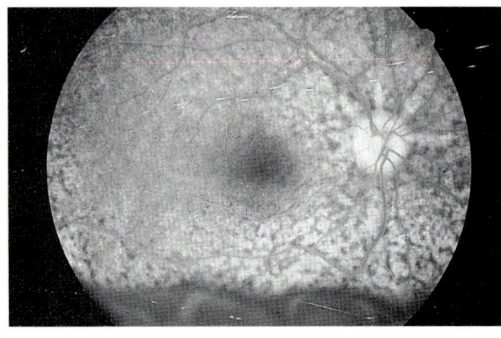
B

All of the following are true *except*

a. B-scan echography is likely to show diffuse choroidal thickening.
b. The untreated natural history is that of progressive, usually bilateral, visual decline.
c. Scleral buckling is likely to be curative.
d. A surgical procedure to thin the sclera is likely to result in resolution of the retinal detachment.

R49 A 23-year-old woman complains of unilateral paracentral scotomas and photopsias. Visual acuity is 20/40 in the left eye, and visual field testing shows enlargement of the physiologic blind spot on the left. Fundus appearance (part A) and fluorescein findings (part B) are shown in the figures. The right eye is normal.

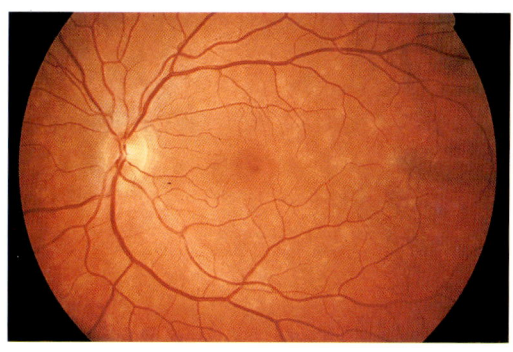 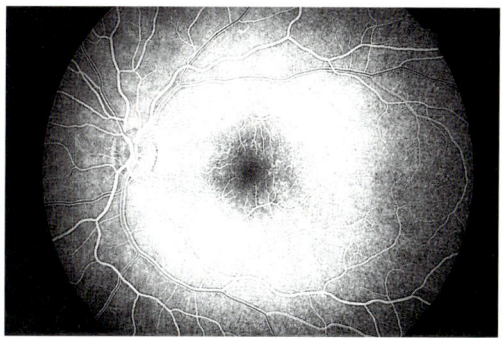

A   B

This clinical presentation is *most* characteristic of

a. idiopathic central serous chorioretinopathy
b. multiple evanescent white dot syndrome
c. acute posterior multifocal placoid pigment epitheliopathy
d. serpiginous choroiditis

R50 A 35-year-old man presents with recurrent bilateral iridocyclitis, sometimes including hypopyon. He reports recurrent genital ulcers and reddish bumps on his skin. Examination reveals the oral ulcers (see the figure, part A) and posterior segment findings (see the figure, part B).

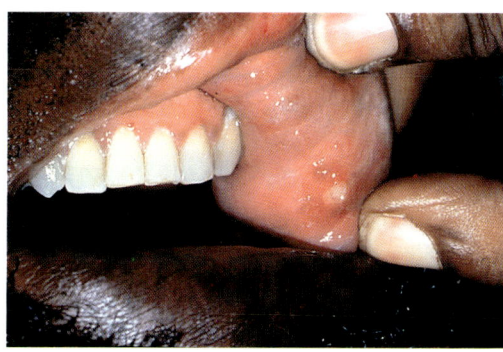 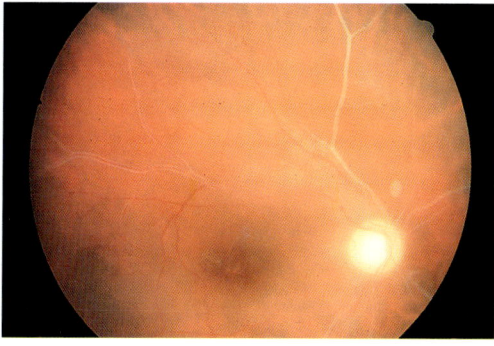

A   B

All of the following are true *except*

a. This disease is most common in the Middle and Far East.
b. Pricking the skin with a needle may help confirm the diagnosis.
c. Immunosuppressive agents are frequently used for treatment of the associated retinal vasculitis.
d. Untreated patients have an excellent prognosis.

SECTION EIGHT

Optics, Refraction, Contact Lens, and Visual Rehabilitation

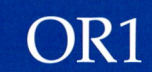
An intraocular lens (IOL) placed in the capsular bag following phacoemulsification and continuous-tear capsulorrhexis has moved axially toward the cornea over the first 6 weeks after surgery as a result of contraction of the capsule. The refractive change that would be expected from the anterior axial movement of an IOL is

a. hyperopic shift
b. no effect
c. myopic shift
d. not determinable

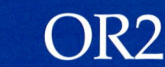
Five years ago, a patient underwent bilateral 16-incision radial keratotomy with a 3 mm optical zone. This patient has now developed 4 mm posterior subcapsular cataracts in each eye. His vision is limited to 20/50 visual acuity OU due to the cataracts, and IOL implantation is planned. The *least* accurate method for determining the corneal K readings to be used for IOL calculation in this patient is

a. manual keratometry
b. automated keratometry
c. calculation of change in refraction with and without a hard contact lens
d. calculation of K readings from preoperative radial keratometry K readings and the change in refraction

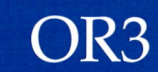
Which of the following statements about antireflection coatings on eyeglasses is true?

a. They are applied by a dipping process.
b. They decrease reflections by producing a matte surface.
c. They work by destructive interference of reflected light.
d. They are always clear and colorless.

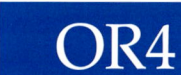
All of the following are indications for planned replacement of soft contact lenses *except*

a. mucus formation and secretions
b. 3 and 9 o'clock staining
c. giant papillary conjunctivitis
d. limbal epithelial hypertrophy

149

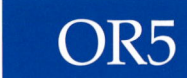

Closed-circuit television systems provide great assistance for many individuals with low vision. Which of the following statements is true?

a. Like many magnification systems, closed-circuit television requires the user to be at a specific distance for proper usage.
b. Closed-circuit television systems have the ability to present black letters on a white background or white letters on a black background. This reverse polarity is useful for patients with photophobia, who prefer to read black letters on a white background.
c. Patients who can no longer benefit from standard magnification systems also cannot be helped with closed-circuit television systems.
d. Many people who successfully use closed-circuit television systems also use other optical aids for specific tasks.

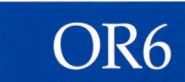

Monocular diplopia, in which the patient sees a ghost image adjacent to the primary image, can arise from any of the following *except*

a. immature cataract
b. age-related maculopathy
c. early keratoconus
d. uncorrected refractive error

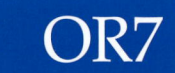

Nine months after successful cryotherapy to a peripheral retinal tear, a patient develops slightly decreased vision in the treated eye and what appears to be 1 prism diopter of vertical diplopia that disappears when either eye is closed. A 1 prism diopter vertical prism, taped to the glasses, immediately relieves the diplopia, but it recurs 10 seconds later. Several trials with additional prisms are similarly unsuccessful, with the diplopia recurring in minutes to hours.

What is the *most* likely cause of the diplopia?

a. a decompensating vertical phoria
b. the top of the bifocal segment covering part of the pupil
c. an epiretinal membrane with vertical foveal dragging and central diplopia
d. monocular diplopia from an early cataract

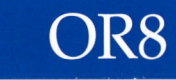

Which of the following intraocular lens designs would be *most* affected by a 15° lens tilt?

a. convexoplano (convex anterior)
b. planoconvex (convex posterior)
c. biconvex
d. meniscus

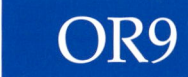

OR9 A 21-year-old male college student ruptured his penetrating keratoplasty incision 3 months ago in his right eye. Although this eye is beginning to stabilize after surgical repair, visual recovery is still incomplete. He reports several episodes of corneal abrasion on his left keratoconic eye.

You might attempt contact lens fitting for the left eye by using

a. disposable soft lens for comfort even though the vision would not be optimal
b. a reusable soft lens for comfort
c. a soft basement lens (reusable or disposable) with a rigid lens on top ("piggyback" system)
d. limited wearing time of a traditional gas-permeable lens

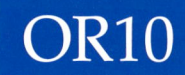

OR10 What trial reading add would be a good initial approximation in a base prescription for a patient who has a distance visual acuity in the range of 20/200?

a. +2.00 D lens
b. +5.00 D lens
c. +10.00 D lens
d. +20.00 D lens

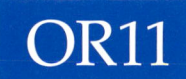

OR11 After cataract surgery with IOL implantation, a patient obtains a new plastic spectacle lens and complains of double vision through the reading segment. Which of the following is the *best* therapeutic approach?

a. Prescribe a slab-off prism based on calculations involving the powers of the pre- and postoperative spectacle lenses.
b. Prescribe a slab-off prism based on measurement of the vertical misalignment in down gaze.
c. Prescribe a reverse-slab prism based on calculations involving the powers of the pre- and postoperative spectacle lenses.
d. Prescribe a reverse-slab prism based on measurement of the vertical misalignment in down gaze.

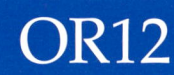

OR12 An aphakic patient with a refraction of +12.00 +3.00 × 180 at a vertex distance of 14 mm is considering a secondary implant. If the secondary implant surgery has no effect on the corneal astigmatism and the postoperative target is emmetropia, the expected postoperative refraction would be

a. plano
b. −1.50 +3.00 × 180
c. −1.50 +3.00 × 90
d. −2.25 +4.50 × 180

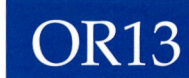

OR13 Which of the following statements about fixed-focus stand magnifiers is true?

a. To reduce peripheral aberrations, the lens is set closer to the page than its focal length. Therefore, a moderate reading add or accommodative effort is required to bring the image into focus.
b. When a patient is using a stand magnifier and a reading add, the combined power of the lens system is that of a simple lens system and can be determined by adding the powers of the add and the magnifier.
c. The field of a stand magnifier is not dependent on the viewing distance.
d. Stand magnifiers are less useful than hand magnifiers for patients who are tremulous.

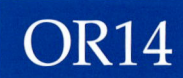

OR14 Which of the following statements about round-top bifocal segments is true?

a. They cause significant image jump on plus lenses but not on minus lenses.
b. They increase image displacement on plus lenses.
c. They are generally preferred over flat-top segments for use on minus lenses.
d. They are generally preferred for use on plus lenses.

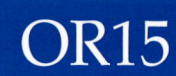

OR15 A 25-year-old patient presents with a refraction of −6.00 D in the right eye with 20/20 visual acuity and −9.00 D in the left eye with 20/200 visual acuity. The visual acuity has decreased in the left eye over the last year because of a traumatic cataract, and the refraction in the right eye has been stable for many years. The patient cannot tolerate contact lenses.

What should the target refraction be for the left eye?

a. plano
b. −0.50 D
c. −1.00 D
d. −4.50 D

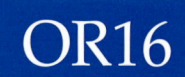

OR16 Which of the following statements about chromatic aberration of prisms, lenses, or the eye is true?

a. It represents a well-known exception to Snell's law, with different angles of refraction occurring with the same angle of incidence.
b. It causes the blue rays to come into focus anterior to the red rays in the eye (closer to the crystalline lens).
c. It is minimized in spectacle lenses by using high-index glass or plastic.
d. It is the basis of the duochrome (red-green) test commonly used for binocular balancing.

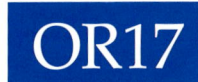

All of the following are good indications for rigid bifocal contact lenses *except*

a. successful monovision (one contact lens at reading refraction and one contact lens at distance refraction)
b. previous successful contact lens wear
c. normal external examination
d. failure of monovision

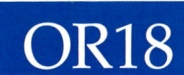

For a physician not currently performing low-vision examinations, what is required to initiate low-vision services in a private office?

a. a well-stocked low-vision cabinet, costing several thousand dollars, containing most of the magnification devices
b. a technician trained in low-vision services
c. a preassembled low-vision kit, costing several hundred dollars, available through retail outlets
d. closed-circuit television aids

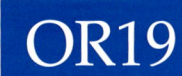

A patient complains of a starburst pattern and haze around lights at night with her pseudophakic eye. Her vision is correctable to 20/50. The pupil dilates to 8 mm, revealing an opacified posterior capsule. A 2 mm Nd:YAG laser posterior capsulotomy is subsequently performed and the patient's visual acuity returns to 20/20. Although her symptoms improve, she still complains of haze and starburst with oncoming headlights at night.

The *most* likely cause is

a. IOL optically damaged with the Nd:YAG laser
b. capsular opening too small for scotopic pupil
c. vitreous floaters in visual axis
d. positioning holes in IOL optic within the capsular opening

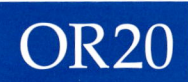

Moving a plus spectacle lens forward (away from the cornea) when viewing a distant object

a. decreases the size of the retinal image
b. cannot be compensated for by an increase in accommodation
c. decreases the effective plus power of the lens
d. will blur objects viewed at intermediate distances

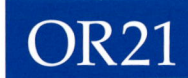 **OR21** A 42-year-old male with a history of severe diabetic retinopathy has had secondary glaucoma and enucleation of his left eye. He presents in your office with an extended-wear aphakic soft lens in place that has not been removed for many months because of lack of family support. The patient's refraction is +11.75 D sphere to correct visual acuity to 20/40. His keratometric readings are spherical, and the mire images are free of distortion. His current soft contact lens corrects his visual acuity to 20/60.

The *best* approach to provide a safer fitting regimen as well as to improve vision would be

a. aphakic spectacles
b. disposable soft contact lens
c. gas-permeable contact lens
d. extended-wear soft contact lens of corrected power

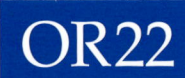 **OR22** A 26-year-old emmetrope with ocular albinism, foveal hypoplasia, and moderate low vision has visual acuities of 20/200 in each eye separately but 20/140 visual acuity binocularly. His preferred reading distance is 8 cm, but he complains of significant eye fatigue and headaches. For near reading performance, the preferred low-vision aid is

a. a +12.00 D aspheric spectacle
b. a +10.00 D prismatic half-eye spectacle
c. a high-add bifocal (+5.00 D) on a plano carrier
d. a hand-held 4× magnifier

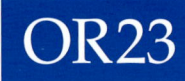 **OR23** An uncorrected bilateral 2.00 D hyperope with an accommodative amplitude of 3.00 D

a. will probably have asthenopic symptoms, even for distance vision
b. will see comfortably at 40 cm with single-vision reading glasses of +1.50 D
c. has a far point 50 cm in front of the eyes
d. has a near point 20 cm in front of the eyes

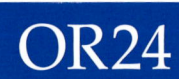 **OR24** A 20.0 D biconvex IOL is tilted 20° about the vertical axis (90°). This situation would result in which of the following spectacle prescriptions if the patient were emmetropic with no lens tilt?

a. $-0.75 -2.00 \times 90$
b. $-0.75 +2.00 \times 90$
c. $+0.75 -2.00 \times 90$
d. $+0.75 +2.00 \times 90$

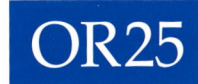

A 68-year-old woman presents with age-related macular degeneration, atrophic foveae with 20/200 visual acuity, +3.50 D of hyperopia, and moderate cataract with heavy vacuoles and mild posterior subcapsular opacities. Regarding the low-vision aspects of cataract surgery in this individual, which of the following is *least* accurate?

a. Worsening of cataract symptoms and functional impairment with increased illumination is common and helps to justify cataract surgery.
b. Leaving the patient aphakic and thus wearing aphakic spectacles will give 25% image magnification and enhance low-vision performance.
c. Selecting IOL power for a −2.50 D target postoperative refraction is functionally preferred over emmetropia.
d. With nuclear sclerosis, the addition of mild posterior subcapsular cataract changes or vacuoles can significantly and disproportionately increase the cataract's effect on functional vision.

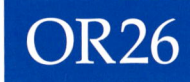

A 31-year-old patient with soft contact lenses in place has an initial corrected visual acuity of 20/400 OU. She wears glasses over her lenses for the rest of her needed correction to provide a best-corrected visual acuity of 20/50 OD and 20/80 OS. She had worn gas-permeable contact lenses 2 years ago but, because of protein buildup, was converted to soft contact lenses. She was advised that her astigmatism would make glasses necessary to refine her vision. Her refraction OD is −16.75 +2.00 × 105 to achieve 20/20 +2; refraction OS is −17.25 +2.00 × 75 to achieve 20/20. Keratometry reveals readings of OD 48.12 D × 93°/46.12 D × 3°, OS 50.00 D × 74°/48.00 D × 164°. Biomicroscopy confirms no corneal thinning. Computerized corneal analysis displays a pattern of with-the-rule astigmatism. The remainder of her ophthalmologic exam is unremarkable.

This patient can *best* be helped visually by

a. keratoconic-design gas-permeable contact lenses
b. reverse-aspheric gas-permeable contact lenses
c. hyperflange gas-permeable contact lenses aided by spectacles
d. hyperflange gas-permeable contact lenses

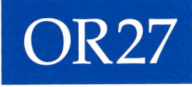

An elderly patient with age-related macular degeneration, parkinsonism, and 20/200 visual acuity in her better eye wishes to keep and wear her current +3.00 D add bifocals and resists holding material closer than 25 cm. The low-vision aid *most* likely to be accepted for near work (such as reading bills or writing) is

a. +4.00 D prismatic half-eye spectacles
b. 4× open-stand magnifier
c. 6× hand-held aspheric magnifier
d. 2.8× loupe hung on the current spectacles over the better eye

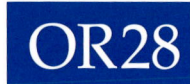

Which of the following is true about an eye that has a spherical cornea but has 1.00 D of with-the-rule simple myopic astigmatism after cataract and IOL surgery?

a. The intraocular lens is undoubtedly tilted about its vertical axis.
b. The astigmatism can be decreased by loosening one or more sutures in the horizontal meridian if the wound has been closed in that manner.
c. The astigmatism can be corrected with a minus cylinder with its axis placed vertically.
d. The patient may not desire any correction of the astigmatism.

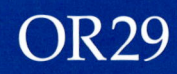

A 43-year-old man underwent bilateral radial keratotomy in 1982. He suffered significant overcorrection of the left eye, creating unacceptable anisometropia, which was corrected by soft contact lenses in both eyes. Neovascularization of two of the superior radial incisions—at the 11 and 1 o'clock positions—occurred in the left eye. Subsequently, large-diameter, rigid gas-permeable lenses were fitted but eventually they were discontinued because of concerns about further superior neovascularization. After discontinuation of these lenses, a circumferential-incision suturing procedure was performed in the left eye in an effort to reduce the patient's residual left hyperopia. This procedure was not successful, and several suture knots are still buried in the stroma. The patient's current refraction OD is $+2.25 - 0.25 \times 151$ to achieve 20/20, and OS is $+8.50 - 0.50 \times 156$ to achieve 20/25. He is an emerging presbyope and is using reading glasses. This patient is a private pilot and needs to maintain binocular vision.

Which of the following nonsurgical options could be used to achieve binocularity?

a. spectacles with less plus correction for the left eye
b. disposable soft contact lenses aided by glasses for residual correction
c. a single soft contact lens for the left eye and reading glasses
d. gas-permeable contact lenses with reverse-curve design aided by reading glasses

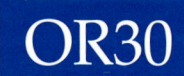

Regarding general low-vision rehabilitation, which of the following is *least* effective?

a. repositioning and enlarging the available visual field using selective prisms
b. increasing angular magnification by moving the object closer to the lens
c. enhancing target contrast by manipulating background color and object saturation
d. augmenting the illumination source with greater wattage and broader-spectrum output

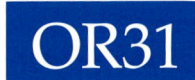 Surgical loupes are designed for a given working distance. This working distance may be

a. increased by omitting habitual myopic correction in the surgeon's glasses
b. increased by adding a plus lens to the front of the loupe
c. increased by adding a plus lens to the rear of the loupe
d. effectively increased by choosing a lower-power loupe with the same nominal working distance

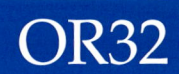 The fabricated add on a −15.00 D pair of spectacles is +2.00. The 45-year-old patient complains that near vision is still blurry. The glasses are measured on a lensmeter with the posterior surface against the lensmeter, and the add is measured to be +1.50 D. Why is the measured add weaker than the prescription?

a. The optician made the add power incorrectly.
b. The effective add is always less than the fabricated add in high-minus glasses.
c. The effective add is always less than the fabricated add in high-plus glasses.
d. Image minification by high-minus lenses causes the effective add and the fabricated add to be different.

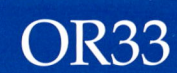 Neutralization of the retinoscopic reflex with the streak retinoscope and trial lenses

a. places the far point of the combination of the patient's eye and the trial lenses at infinity
b. locates the far point of the patient
c. is not affected by the patient's accommodation
d. places the circle of least confusion on the retina

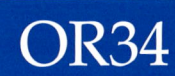 When a patient cannot read the 20/400 line on a standard eye chart at the standard distance, what should the ophthalmologist do?

a. Measure the visual acuity by having the patient count fingers at the maximum distance possible.
b. Obtain a numeric visual acuity score by testing with a chart at a closer distance.
c. Record the visual acuity as "less than 20/400."
d. Record the visual acuity as "hand movements only."

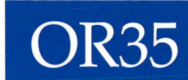 Because of the large optical corrections required for extremely high-myopic patients, glasses have poor cosmetic appearance and limited function (see the figure). Yet the manufacturing limitations of contact lenses also make them challenging for realizing the full visual potential.

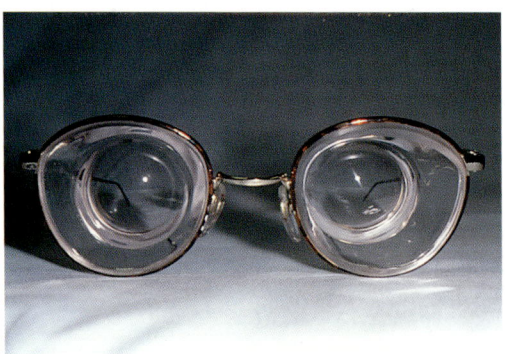

An example of best design and usage would be

a. spherical soft contact lenses aided by glasses
b. tinted soft contact lenses aided by glasses
c. tinted gas-permeable contact lenses with special edge design
d. hybrid contact lenses with rigid center and soft skirt

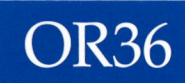 A patient who wears rigid gas-permeable contact lenses has developed bilateral posterior subcapsular cataracts that have decreased the visual acuity to 20/60 OU. Keratometry readings and axial lengths are measured for IOL calculations. The K readings are spherical at 45.00 D for each eye with no irregularity; the axial lengths are 23.5 mm. The contact lenses were fitted elsewhere so pre–contact lens K readings are unavailable.

For this patient, it would be appropriate to

a. use the present spherical K readings and recommended IOL powers
b. discontinue the contact lenses for 24 hours and repeat K readings
c. discontinue the contact lenses for 1 week, repeat K readings, and use the average of the two measurements
d. discontinue the contact lenses and repeat K readings weekly until stable (two consecutive measurements the same)

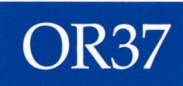 A 75-year-old man has a stable but profound reduction in vision, having previously developed subfoveal choroidal neovascular membranes in both eyes. His best-corrected visual acuity is 20/480 in each eye. A central visual field defect with a diameter of approximately 7° is noted in both eyes. The peripheral visual field is intact.

All of the following statements are true *except*

a. The patient may be able to read continuous text by using a video magnifier (closed-circuit television).
b. The patient's ability to use residual vision may be improved by training in eccentric viewing techniques.
c. A +10.00 D add would be the minimum add necessary to resolve 20/40 near vision (newsprint size, Jaeger 3, or 1M in metric system).
d. The patient may experience difficulty with negotiating street crossings and have other mobility concerns.

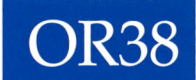

A patient who wants to be fitted with contact lenses has a spectacle refraction of −8.00 +3.00 × 90 bilaterally and K readings of 45.00 D × 90°/42.50 D × 180° bilaterally. Which type of lens would be *most* appropriate?

a. a bitoric, rigid gas-permeable contact lens
b. a soft, nontoric, disposable contact lens
c. a spherical, rigid gas-permeable contact lens
d. a toric soft contact lens without prism ballast

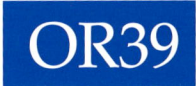

An 8-year-old phakic boy has a quiet eye following repair of traumatic corneal laceration. His fellow eye is emmetropic. An aspheric gas-permeable contact lens has been suggested to correct the moderate amount of irregular astigmatism of the injured eye.

Which of the following would be a reasonable choice for providing best visual acuity with adequate protection for both eyes?

a. spectacles only; too young for contact lens
b. soft toric contact lens with ultraviolet protection
c. gas-permeable contact lens during school hours only
d. ultraviolet-absorbing gas-permeable contact lens worn with sports goggles for outside activities

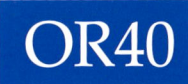

A 75-year-old man with atrophic age-related macular degeneration has a visual acuity of 20/70 in both eyes. As a retired newspaper editor, he expresses great frustration with his inability to read the newspaper; he can see the characters on a page but has difficulty making the letters into words and words into sentences. After completing a line of text, he has difficulty finding the next line at the left margin; he frequently finds he is rereading the same line or has missed a line of text. His reading rate is too slow to make reading enjoyable. He has tried using magnifiers but they have not helped much.

The *most* likely cause of his reading difficulty is

a. early dementia
b. ring scotoma surrounding fixation
c. insufficient magnification
d. a poor attitude

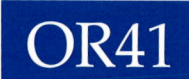**OR41** Which low-vision enhancement technique would be expected to offer the *greatest* benefit for the patient in Question OR40?

a. enhancing magnification by using loupes for near tasks
b. adjusting image contrast with a closed-circuit television that uses reverse-polarity letter projection and computer-sharpened image enhancements
c. increasing illumination with a broad-spectrum fluorescent light
d. arranging for Library of Congress books on tape for auditory access to printed material

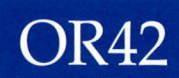**OR42** A patient with age-related macular degeneration has developed nuclear sclerotic cataracts. The best-corrected visual acuity in each eye is counting fingers at 1 foot, but with the potential acuity meter the retinal acuity is 20/200. Current spectacles and best refraction are nearly plano. The *best* target for the postoperative refraction would be

a. target +8.00 D so that the patient can get magnification from the high-plus glasses
b. target plano to give the best-uncorrected visual acuity
c. target −3.00 D to provide near vision with no significant effect on distance acuity
d. use negative IOL to create a Galilean telescope with high-plus glasses

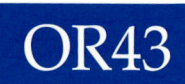**OR43** After cataract and IOL surgery, an eye has a refraction of −1.00 +1.50 × 90 and K readings of 43.00 D/43.00 D. The astigmatism may be caused by

a. decentration of the IOL
b. an eccentric pupil
c. a tilted IOL
d. a tilted retina

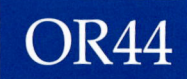**OR44** A 6-week-old patient with monocular aphakia has a correction of +18.00 D at a vertex distance of 12 mm. Even though keratometry is not available for this spherical eye, you want to proceed with contact lens fitting for visual rehabilitation.

Which of the following lens powers *best* meets the optical power requirements?

a. +26.00 D
b. +23.00 D
c. +18.00 D
d. +19.00 D

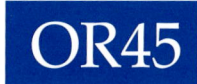

OR45 An 82-year-old woman who is undergoing cataract and IOL surgery in her right eye has a preoperative refraction of +3.00 D sphere = 20/60 OD and +3.50 D sphere = 20/25 OS. Postoperatively, the refraction OD is −2.50 +1.00 × 80, yielding a visual acuity of 20/20. On receiving the new corrective lens, she may experience difficulty from any of the following problems *except*

a. diplopia on side gaze
b. diplopia on down gaze
c. monocular diplopia
d. unequal image sizes

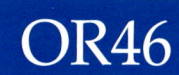

OR46 A patient with severe bilateral cataracts has been emmetropic in both eyes most of his life. He undergoes uneventful cataract surgery with implantation of a +20.0 D biconvex IOL in his first eye. The final correction in the first eye is 20/20 with a −0.50 D refraction. Surgery is performed on the second eye 2 months later with implantation of the same power and style of IOL. On the first day postoperatively the patient shows a visual acuity of counting fingers at 3 feet with no correction but refracts to 20/40 with a −12.00 D sphere.

The *most* likely explanation for this large refractive surprise is

a. mismeasured axial length
b. mismeasured K reading
c. lens optic is implanted upside down
d. mislabeled IOL

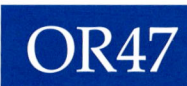

OR47 Fluctuating visual function after radial keratotomy is seen because of any of the following *except*

a. fluctuating macular edema
b. a decentered optical zone
c. a small optical zone
d. fluctuating refractive error

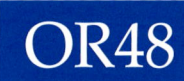

OR48 A first-time wearer of gas-permeable contact lenses complains of blurred vision at the 2-week follow-up visit. Further discussion reveals that visual acuity levels seem to fall as the day progresses and that the lenses are difficult to remove. The patient reports that her eyes are slightly red at the end of the day but that this injection is gone by morning. Slit-lamp observation reveals faint 3 and 9 o'clock staining but is otherwise unremarkable. The lenses appear to meet normal criteria for a satisfactory fit.

Which of the following would be a reasonable procedure?

a. Do not alter the fit, as this is a novice wearer and the absence of significant findings suggests waiting for further follow-up.
b. Switch the patient to soft contact lenses to satisfy comfort and vision issues.
c. Contact lens adhesion may be occurring late in the day; parameter changes should be made.
d. Enlarge the diameter of the lens by 0.4 mm to enhance the stability of vision.

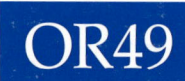

Which of the following is true when macular disease results in loss of foveal function and subsequently produces a dense central scotoma?

a. A preferred retinal locus for fixation will naturally and reliably occur in a paracentral location.
b. Letter recognition is not possible.
c. Color perception is lost.
d. Diplopia is likely to be experienced during training in the use of magnifiers.

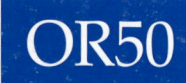

Before cataract surgery with IOL placement in the left eye, a patient's glasses measure +1.00 +0.50 × 30 = 20/25 OD and plano +2.50 × 120 = 20/50 OS. Postoperatively, the spectacle refraction of the left eye is +1.00 sphere = 20/20+.

With the new lens in place, the patient is likely to complain of

a. monocular diplopia in the spectacle-corrected left eye
b. decreased visual field in the left eye
c. distortion of vision in the left eye under monocular conditions
d. orientation problems